The Nest
in the
Stream

D1009951

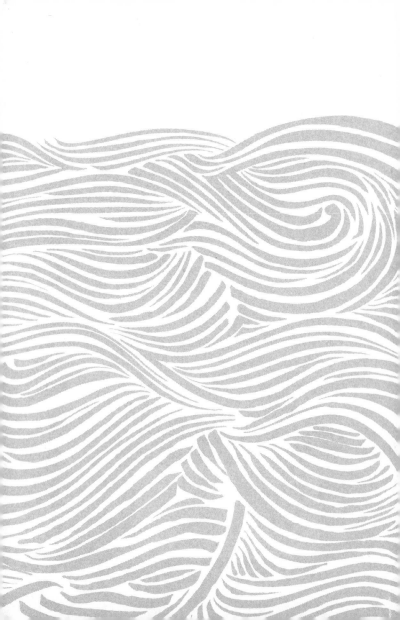

"In a quiet, gradually illuminating way Michael Kearney introduces us to a few key spiritual and emotional discoveries he made during his work as a palliative care doctor and as a novice in Native American rites of passage. The writing is clear and beautiful, the lessons easily present to the mind, and the vision truly inspiring. I loved reading this book and know that its wisdom will stay with me, lightening the burden."

—Thomas Moore, author of *Care of the Soul*

Received on
FEB 10 2020
Green Lake Library

NO LONGER PROPERTY OF
SEATTLE PUBLIC LIBRARY

"In this dear book, Michael yet again takes us deeper, closer. He nudges us to see that to understand someone is to care for them. Yes, love them. This book is most directly about the cautions and craft of caregiving. And it is about receiving too, as though by necessity these come together. This is the sweet reciprocal loop that Michael has been pointing out to me for many years now and I'm so glad he's offered us more stories and intimacies to reify this subtly potent point. For all its quietness, this book is full of brave explorations just beyond the line of familiarity. And since he dares to look and see—we can too."

—B.J. Miller MD, Zen Hospice Project, presenter of 2015 TED talk *What Really Matters at The End of Life*

"Kearney's work is deep, thorough, risky, elegant and poetic. He is an exemplar for all those who come to realize that self-healing is a necessary condition for helping others to be healed. It is a win-win bargain. This is a warrior's path, redefining the meaning of manhood and bravery and engaging the deepest and most challenging purposes of life."

—Edward Bastian, PhD, Director Spiritual Paths Foundation

"Michael Kearney has written a wonderful book. I read it in one sitting and was left with a new sense of the preciousness of life and present again to the longing to make a difference in other people's lives that motivates whole person care. It should be mandatory reading for all medical students and physicians in practice. But its interest is not limited to people with medical expertise. I find it hard to imagine a person who would not enjoy and benefit from this soul-nurturing book."

—Tom Hutchinson MD, Medical Director McGill Center for Whole Person Care, McGill University, Montreal

"Michael Kearney's *The Nest in the Stream* is a deeply moving account of the author's search for healing in lives filled with pain: his patients', his own, and the world's. Throughout, his relationship with nature is paramount and profound. He finds his way into its inner reaches, and it ripples through the fine-grained net of his sparsely elegant poetic prose. The reader is grateful for the gift of this singular book: its sure and subtle vision as well as its genius for finding connectivity everywhere, indeed for realizing that one is this very connectivity. In the end, the reader comes to know that being at one with 'all our relations' is the heart of healing."

—Edward S. Casey, Distinguished Professor of Philosophy,
SUNY at Stony Brook; Distinguished Visiting Faculty,
Pacifica Graduate Institute

"I started the book and could not put it down for three hours. It weaves between clinical experiences and philosophical and spiritual insights of some of Kearney's previous works and personal biography like a Celtic knot. It is a unique form of biography that bridges the personal with the universal."

—James Morley, PhD, Professor of Clinical Psychology,
Ramapo College of New Jersey

"You and I, and our home, this threatened planet, share a common journey through pain, in a quest for healing and wholeness. Whatever our perception, each of us is involved as both sufferer and caregiver. In this sensitive, wise and wondrously revealing memoir, physician and wounded healer Michael Kearney plumbs the depths of his personal path while drawing on a galaxy of inspired teachers. This is a profoundly important book."

—Balfour Mount MD, Emeritus Eric M. Flanders Chair of Palliative
Medicine, McGill University, Montreal

"I always know when a book has entered into my soul when I find myself drawing on it frequently in my clinical practice and personal life. This is such a book! I am sure it will make a deep impact on others in the helping professions and those who care about themselves and others."

—Mary L.S. Vachon, PhD, RN, Adjunct Professor, Department of
Psychiatry and Dalla Lana School of Public Health, University of Toronto

"Beneath, above, beside, and inside the life we think we are living, lays another life, often cast out of our awareness. This wider life is not only our *experience* of being held by nature, but the fact of our being part of nature. Michael Kearney brings this other life into focus as he shares lucid stories of experiencing interconnection with other-than-human nature. As a wounded healer, Kearney awakens us to how we often deal with grief and suffering. He offers pathways to standing in our wider home, as we turn toward suffering with an open heart."

—Mary Watkins, Chair MA, PhD, Depth Psychology Program,
Pacifica Graduate Institute, Santa Barbara

"There is no one in the field of medicine and healing I respect more than Michael Kearney, MD. Whenever a book of his appears it is a reason for celebration. But when he writes about suffering in an ever-deepening way until in the end of the book one feels one has traveled to the underworld and back, one is awestruck. His words have the power to confront loneliness and make us feel embedded in the social and natural world around us. This is a story of the suffering of humans and of Nature, and of a doctor who admits his fear of pain yet who doesn't flinch. Anyone who has ever suffered will find this book a revelation. I sure did!"

—Robert Bosnak, PsyA, Jungian psychoanalyst,
author of *Tracks in the Wilderness of Dreaming*

"Some seeds need to be scarified—cracked open in the grit of a creek-bed, say, making them amenable to water—before they can become seedlings, then saplings, then great, shade-making trees. This is the story of such a journey. A magnanimous, gently wise, at times wrenchingly vulnerable account of one man's gritty 'heart-work' done for the sake of all our relations. Read it and be cracked open. Read it to remember things you perhaps didn't know you forgot. Read it to root deeper into this earth and into your life. Read it and be returned."

—Teddy Macker, author of *This World*

MICHAEL KEARNEY, MD

FOREWORD BY *Joanna Macy*

The Nest
in the
Stream

Lessons from Nature
on Being with Pain

PARALLAX
PRESS

BERKELEY, CALIFORNIA

Parallax Press

P.O. Box 7355

Berkeley, California 94707

parallax.org

Parallax Press is the publishing division

of Plum Village Community of Engaged Buddhism, Inc.

Copyright © 2018 by Michael Kearney

All rights reserved

Printed in The United States of America

Cover and text design by Jess Morphew

Cover and interior art © CPD-Lab/iStock /Getty Images Plus

Author Photo © Stephanie Baker

ISBN: 978-1-946764-00-3

Library of Congress Cataloging-in-Publication Data

Names: Kearney, Michael (Physician), author.

Title: The nest in the stream : lessons from nature on being with pain / by
  Michael Kearney.

Description: Berkeley, CA : Parallax Press, [2018] | Includes bibliographical
  references.

Identifiers: LCCN 2017042774 (print) | LCCN 2017044445 (ebook) | ISBN
  9781946764010 (Ebook) | ISBN 9781946764003 (pbk.)

Subjects: | MESH: Pain Management--psychology | Faith Healing--psychology |
  Spiritual Therapies | Nature | Personal Narratives

Classification: LCC RZ401 (ebook) | LCC RZ401 (print) | NLM WL 704.6 | DDC
  615.8/52--dc23

LC record available at https://lccn.loc.gov/2017042774

1 2 3 4 5 / 22 21 20 19 18

To my grandsons Elliot, Alex, and Finn,
and to all the grandchildren

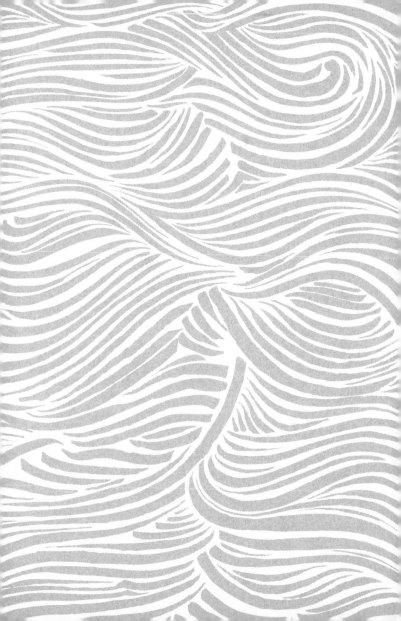

If we surrendered
to Earth's intelligence
we could rise up rooted, like trees.

Rainer Maria Rilke

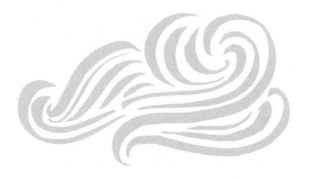

Contents

Author's Note 15

Foreword 17

BY JOANNA MACY

ONE

Beginnings

MONDAY EVENING, MAY | 22

A SEARCH FOR HEALING | 34

RELATING TO PAIN | 62

TWO

Seven Stories of Nature Connection

FIRST: COLMAN'S WELL | 76

SECOND: THE OTHER SIDE OF THE ROAD | 80

THIRD: THE LAND | 84

FOURTH: THE NEST IN THE STREAM | 96

FIFTH: UP ON THE HILL | 107

SIXTH: THE TREE OF LIFE | 116

SEVENTH: POLARIS | 128

THREE

————

Endings

MONDAY EVENING, JUNE | 136

LESSONS FROM NATURE | 140

A STORY ENDS | 142

INTO THE DEEPER STREAM | 153

Notes 164

About the Author 169

Acknowledgments 170

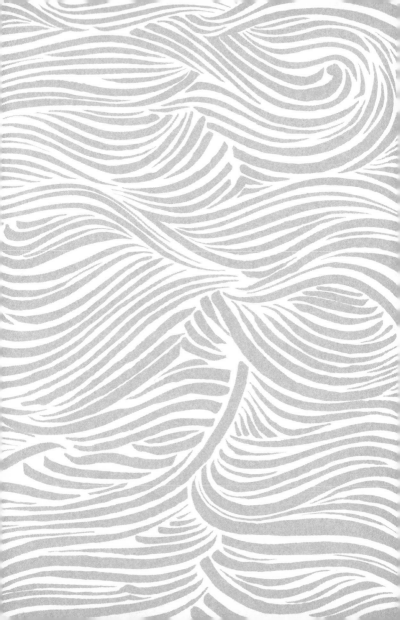

Author's Note

While I am grateful to many individuals for their help in the writing of this book, I am especially indebted to my Native American teachers, Wolf and Lisa Wahpepah. They have welcomed me into their community and given me permission to share what I have learned. I hope I have recorded their words and described their culture with sensitivity and accuracy. That is my intention. I am grateful for the trust they placed in me.

Wolf and Lisa have made clear to me that the particular ways they perform ceremony, which I describe in the book, reflect the teachings they received from their elders. They emphasize that among the more than five hundred tribal nations in North America, there are many legitimate and varied ways of conducting Native ceremonies. Another Native elder, having read the manuscript, made the same point to me. She spoke of how the land itself shapes the ceremony, and put it like this: "There are as many ways of performing ceremony as there are differences in the landscape."

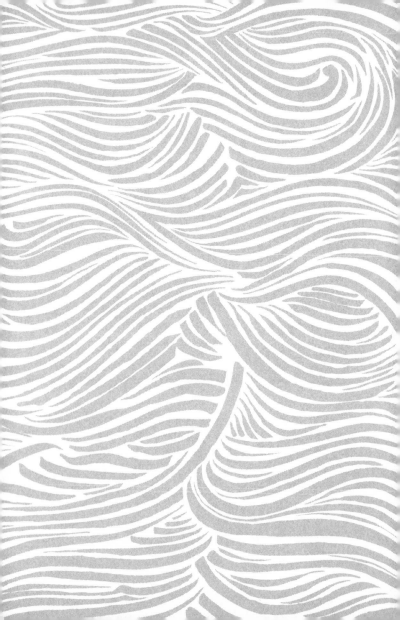

Foreword

BY JOANNA MACY

The Nest in the Stream is the story of a man who dared to face his moral discomfort as a physician and question the medical model of his training—even his own suitability for that profession—when he realized the inadequacy of what he had been taught in the face of his patients' uncontrollable pain and suffering. The book soon moves beyond his personal story to examine how we relate to our world in this time he calls a "tsunami of suffering." It also shows us how life comes to meet us when we are not afraid to be present to that pain. So the journey described here is a journey for each of us.

The query that leads Dr. Michael Kearney on his quest is *how to be with our pain*. I recognize it well. It is the persistent question that has beckoned and teased me over the last fifty years of my engagement in issues of social and ecological justice. It gave rise to the experiential group process called The Work That Reconnects, whose seeds I have helped to sow in many lands. It is a question we need not so much to answer as to stand before it; indeed, it is crucial that we do this because we have become artists of avoidance. That avoidance takes countless familiar forms from busyness and distraction to intellectual debate and obsessions with self-betterment. But we

are not terminally lost in our escapism, for—I am convinced—
our deepest longing is to rejoin our world, open to the company
of our brother-sister beings, and let that larger life be our guide
as it thrums through us.

I rejoice that this book carries so clearly the voice of the man
himself—his keen but gentle attention, his unassuming fidelity
to his own experience. This is how I came to know Michael
Kearney when, some half dozen years ago, he began taking part
in interactive seminars of The Work That Reconnects. Since
then his reflections and queries have enriched my own.

In this book, as in our conversations, he shares life-
changing moments in nature and in traditional practices—
Native American, Celtic, Buddhist—and how these moments
transform his life as a physician and, more broadly, his life in
the world. In so doing, he describes his experiences, but he does
not prescribe them. And because he is not trying to persuade or
convince, we open ourselves to these experiences; we let them
combine and interweave with our own.

As I read over this exquisitely crafted book, I realize that it
is offering us a hero's journey for our time. As Joseph Campbell
has written, the hero/heroine must descend below the surface of
conventional life and confront—even embrace—the shadow or
monster lurking in the subliminal depths before returning with
greater insight to the challenges and achievements that await.

Foreword

As a physician and as a deeply reflective human being, Michael Kearney leads us farther. He shows us that, in addition to the greater presence of heart and mind we gain from having embraced the pain we had not known how to tolerate, something more occurs. Something new emerges. An answer comes. It comes through nature in living forms—in a robin, a wolf, a covey of ladybugs, a cottonwood tree, the North Star. We need not be surprised: both the scientific and the spiritual revolutions ushering us into the Third Millennium reveal that our Earth is alive. We are not alone here. We are invited back into the pulsing give and take of life itself. If we dare to be real with what we feel, we rediscover the larger being we live within, and enter once more the Great Reciprocity at the heart of the universe.

Berkeley, California
September 2017

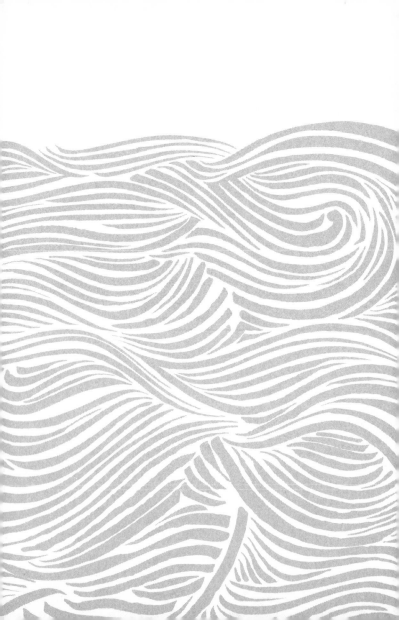

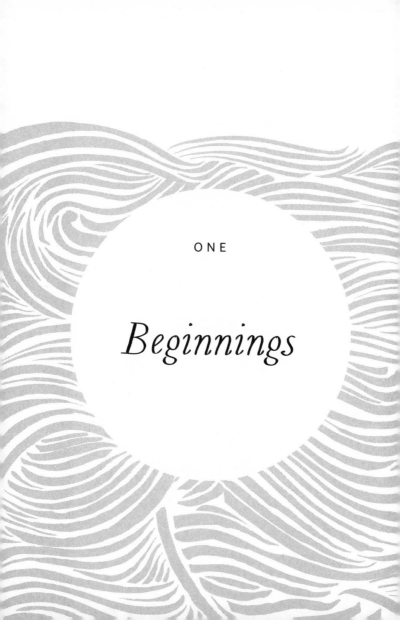

ONE

Beginnings

MONDAY EVENING, MAY

As I go into Ben's hospital room, it is dark; the window blinds are closed. Ben has advanced cancer of the bowel. He is thirty years old and not doing well. He will finish his latest round of chemotherapy this afternoon and then he will go home. He has lost ten pounds in the past two weeks, even though he says he has been eating fairly well. I ask him how he is doing. He says his colostomy has not worked since yesterday morning and that his belly feels tight. He looks tired and I can tell from how he is moving about in his bed that he is in pain.

Just nine months ago, Ben was diagnosed with locally invasive rectal cancer. I was asked to see him as the physician with the palliative care team in the hospital. We had been consulted by Ben's oncologist to try to help him with his pain and to offer emotional support to him and his family as they struggled to cope with his new and serious diagnosis.

When I met Ben and his mother for the first time, Ben was in a room on the oncology floor. I entered his room and found him lying on his side; his rectal pain was so bad that he could not lie flat. I recall how he looked on that first visit—his bright brown eyes, his young bearded face, and the intricate, colorful tattoos on both his arms—and I remember how his mother, Juanita, was sitting at his bedside, her face full of sadness and concern. Ben appeared so strong and well. What had struck me most was his vibrancy, his openness, his gentle directness. He had welcomed my involvement in his care. I had felt happy to meet him.

Unfortunately, since then, things had gone badly for Ben. Despite surgery and first- and second-line chemotherapy, his tumor had recurred and spread throughout his pelvis. He went to Los Angeles for a second surgical opinion and was told that no further surgery was possible. He had had multiple readmissions to the hospital since then for chemotherapy and symptom control.

This current admission had been to start third-line chemotherapy, but afterward his discharge was delayed until now because of severe pelvic pain and other symptoms, which have only recently started to settle down. Ben is due to go home this evening to his grandparents' house. He had moved in to look after them prior to being diagnosed with cancer. His grandfather was very ill himself with end-stage heart disease and had recently been enrolled in hospice care. His grandmother had kidney failure and was on dialysis.

Ben had often spoken to me about his granddad. They are very close. He told me that when he had first received his cancer diagnosis, his grandfather had prayed that he could take on Ben's suffering for him.

A little while ago, Ben's nurse had told me that she had just heard his granddad's condition had deteriorated. She did not know if he was aware that his grandfather was close to death. This could affect his discharge plan.

I ask Ben if he has had news from home. He says no. I tell him I had heard that his granddad is not doing so well and that I wanted him to be aware of this so he will not be surprised when he gets home.

"I'll cheer him up," Ben replies. "Last time when I got home and he saw me, it cheered him up."

"You will, Ben," I say with as much conviction as I can muster. "You will cheer him up." I say goodbye to Ben for now and tell him that the nurse with our community palliative care program will call him tomorrow to make sure he's doing okay. I tell him that I look forward to seeing him when he comes back in two weeks for his next round of chemo.

Despite all his difficulties, Ben has big plans for the future. Recently, he told me that even though he had had a job with a delivery company before becoming ill, his real passion is working with wood. For a few moments, his face lit up as he described different types of timber and shared his plans to open a wood shop with a friend when he is well again. He has not given up hope. He so wants to get well and carry on with being a thirty-year-old.

I have been working with patients like Ben for as long as I have been a doctor. While it can be challenging to control pain such as his, there is always something to do—a dose adjustment here, a new medication there, another line of treatment to explore—and I am grateful for the advances in pain management and interdisciplinary teamwork that have made such a difference for patients like Ben. Finding medical answers is not the problem. The real challenge is something deeper, something more subtle, pervasive, and intractable: those elements of human anguish that lurk within and around and beyond the physical pain, the nonphysical dimensions of pain that do not have an easy fix. That is what I have seen for some days now in the dark rings under Ben's eyes and in his flat expression as he lies in his dim-lit, shuttered room. My medical training had done nothing to prepare me for such distress.

I think of Ben as I am driving home. I notice a hollowness at the center of my chest and realize I am feeling saddened and impotent. I care deeply about him and wish I could do more to help. I feel frustrated with the Western model of medicine, which has so little to offer here, notwithstanding its great achievements and its self-confidence to the point of arrogance. Despite some temporary successes along the way, at some more fundamental level I know that we, his team of clinicians, are failing Ben. Yes, we have eased his pain, but he wants more than this. He wants his health back. He wants his youth back. He wants his life back. Although no one has said so directly, it's looking increasingly unlikely that we are going to be able to achieve this for him.

But there is another kind of failure and a deeper disappointment here. Even though he is surrounded by people who care about him, I sense that Ben feels utterly alone in his suffering. And while his emotional solitude is probably in part a voluntary withdrawal, compounded by the traumatic effects of treatment and the pain of his disease, I suspect that it is mostly because of the uncertainty and grief he is living with. I am acutely aware that what is needed here is not a scalpel or another pill. I long, as one human being to another, to reach out to Ben in his isolation.

When I arrive home, our family dogs, Lenka, an English springer spaniel, and Lucy, a Chihuahua-mix, give me their usual enthusiastic welcome. I take them for their evening walk along the quiet tree-lined roads close to where we live. It's a hot September afternoon. As the dogs sniff around, I linger in the shade and listen to the bird song. I notice a white-breasted nuthatch and watch as he walks along the underside of an oak branch, all the while hunting for insects in the fissures of the bark.

When I get back to the house, I feed the dogs. I look at today's text messages from my daughters and the pictures of the day's activities of my little grandson. I send off a brief reply and begin to get my things together for the Native American sweat lodge I am planning to attend this evening.

I have been attending these ceremonies for more than ten years now. They have become a spiritual lifeline for me and are something I look forward to each week. This way of prayer has become my "church," not in the sense of a religious belief system, but as an Earth-based practice that feeds my spiritual hunger in ways that my root tradition of Roman Catholicism no longer does.

I eat a quick supper and leave a note for my wife, Radhule, who is still at work. I get into my car and begin the one-hour drive south, hoping I won't be delayed by the rush-hour traffic.

As I arrive, I notice that the willow-frame structure of the lodge has already been dressed with canvas tarps, old blankets, and comforters. People are gathering around the fire. Wolf Wahpepah, the water pourer of the sweat lodge and its spiritual leader, is sitting on the ground to the north of the lodge, calling any newcomers to join him. His wife, Lisa, stands nearby, talking to a friend. For more than twenty years they have made these ways of prayer available to whomever comes their way.

I approach the fireplace and look around to see who is there. There are men and women, young and old, Natives and non-Natives. Some are sitting alone, while others are standing side-by-side facing the fire as they chat. A young couple have brought their little baby and are introducing her to everyone. A group of newcomers are now sitting with Wolf in a circle on the ground. He is talking to them quietly about this way of prayer and telling them what to expect in the ceremony. My awkwardness soon fades, and I quickly feel at home in this diverse and welcoming gathering.

To strengthen my prayers, I go to take some tobacco from the stone bowl on the ground. I hold the tobacco to my heart and close my eyes as I think about what I want to pray for this evening. I sit down and look at the sacred fire, blazing logs surrounding the "stone people," the lava stones that are at the heart of the ceremony. I notice that I am full of my concern for Ben. For a moment, I see his gaunt young face. There's a crack between two burning pieces of wood through which I glimpse a glowing, orange-red rock. I step forward and give my tobacco offering to the flames.

Wolf has stood up now and is calling us together. "Relatives, the fire-keeper informs me that the stones are ready. It's time to change into your sweat clothes, take a final drink of water if you want to, and then let's crawl inside."

As I approach the lodge, the firekeeper is by the door holding some burning white sage. The sage smoke purifies the individual and the area around them. I fan the smoke towards my face and chest, get down on the ground on my hands and knees, and crawl to the opening of the lodge where I touch my forehead to the earth. As I do so, I say the greeting, *"For all my relations!"* Wolf replies, "Welcome, relative!" I crawl inside and move, clockwise, "sun-wise," into the dark.

"Bring us the stones!" Wolf says as Lisa leads us in a song to welcome the lava stones, "the grandfathers," who arrive one at a time, glowing red. The doorman uses deer antlers to catch each stone and carefully place it in the fire pit at the center of the lodge. All the while, we are singing a song that welcomes the stone people as friends. One at a time, Lisa drops sacred herbs on the stones. As the fragrant smoke rises, someone close to the stone pit reaches for a handful of smoke and rubs it into his hair.

Wolf calls for the water and the firekeeper passes in a bucket, full to the brim. Wolf touches the base of the bucket to the stones and says, "Water is life," then he rests it on the ground, takes the ladle in his hand, and turns toward the stones. He gives thanks to the Creator for these ways of prayer and for our very lives this day. He sings and prays as he pours water on the stones and the lodge begins to fill with "the breath of the stone people." He talks to us about these grandfathers, "the oldest living beings on the planet." He says that the natural state of the stones is gray, which is how they were when they were found on the desert floor, but that this is not their "original state." Their original state is glowing red, which is how they are when they are born. In the fire they once again burn red and bright. Wolf says that our spirits also have that same quality of brightness when we come into the world but that living in the world and being subject to negativity, over time, can dim our spirit.

"This negativity is not ours," he tells us. "Ours is that original bright spirit. By building the fire, we help the grandfathers to return to their original state. Then, when they come into the lodge, they remember what we did for them and they return the favor. They bring us back to our original state. This is why the sweat lodge is called a 'purification ceremony,' because it washes off that negativity."

As we sit in the break between the first and second of the four parts or rounds of the ceremony, sounds of hissing and bubbling come up from the stone pit. Wolf talks about how the first people prayed in this way before they had conversational language or song. "The original songs in the lodge were the natural sounds of the ceremony that the medicines make, a language that our minds don't understand but our hearts and spirits do. Being in here is not primarily about what words we use. It's about allowing our spirits to mingle with all the helping spirits of the lodge. It's about remembering how to pray." After a pause, he adds, "Prayer is not about what we say or do. Prayer is a state of being. Whenever we're in the state of being that is prayer, everything we say or do is prayer."

Wolf calls for more stones and, as they are brought in, he invites people to offer a prayer, if they would like to do so. A young woman talks about how she is having a hard time with panic attacks and prays for help. She signals that she is finished with her prayer by saying the word, "Aho!" Others quietly echo, "Aho!" in understanding and support.

I think of Ben. I see that he is dying, even though I hope he is not. Ben doesn't want to die, yet I sense, at some level, he realizes what is happening, and this is fueling a deeper pain: the pain that I have not been able to reach. I feel so powerless. I wish I could do more.

The sweat is pouring down my body now and dripping from my hands. I let it carry all that I am feeling for Ben in its flow. As if he heard me, Wolf says, "We can bring our pain to the stone people and offer it to them. Like the water we pour, we can let our pain go to the stones. Just as the sweat flows from our bodies, we allow our pain to fall on the Earth. The Earth doesn't judge our offering as positive or negative, good or bad; it doesn't put a value on it. Mother Earth just receives whatever we offer her as energy. She takes that energy back into her body and transforms it into pure life force ..." As I listen to Wolf's words, something in me quiets, listens, remembers. I sense that I am receiving a teaching I already know, yet am searching for. I make a silent prayer for Ben, for his deepest healing, whatever happens, and I pray for his family.

Wolf hands Lisa the drum and asks her to lead us in song. He continues to pour the water as the drumbeat begins. The heat intensifies to a point where my face is stinging. My feet are now a puddle of mud. I feel cramped and uncomfortable and my neck is strained from bending beneath the willow beam that's pressing against the back of my head. I try to wriggle into a more comfortable position in the tiny space without bothering my neighbors. Then Lisa begins to sing. I recognize the song and I join in. I give myself completely to the singing. As I do, I notice that a quality of spaciousness and stillness has come into my awareness. I am singing with all my heart and I am silently watching myself singing with all my heart. The song ends and Wolf says, "All together!" With one voice we call out, *"For all my relations!"* The firekeeper, hearing this as a signal, raises the flap and allows cool air inside.

The fourth and final round begins with Lisa singing a song of gratitude. As I join in, I suddenly understand something I once heard her say about the transformative power of the sweat lodge ceremony. She had talked about the "energy transfer" that happens between "the sacreds" in the ceremony—the stones, the water, the songs, the prayers—and us human "two-leggeds." I flash back to how I had been feeling when I got here this evening. I had arrived full of the stresses of my day at work and worries about Ben, feeling tense and shut down.

Now we are approaching the end of the ceremony. The stones that were red at the start of this round have turned gray, having been cooled by the water poured on them. As I watch this, I am aware of what feels like a glow at the center of my chest. Where there had been heaviness, there is now lightness and warmth, and a sense of being in the right place.

As the final song finishes, Wolf talks to us about what will happen next. He says, "In a few moments we'll crawl outside. I encourage you to stay in silence for a little while as you offer each other a drink of water. Act as you would after waking up from a powerful medicine dream." He finishes by saying, "In crawling in here tonight, we crawled into the womb of Mother Earth. Now, as we crawl out, we do so as brothers and sisters."

Together we cry out, *"For all my relations!"*

A SEARCH FOR HEALING

Looking back on my journey as a healer, I see that the tracks leading to where I am in the later stages of my career are not in a straight line. I can relate well to poet Rainer Maria Rilke's words, "I live my life in widening circles."[1]

What came before what I learned along the way about the nature of pain and suffering and healing is still there, but now there is more. There have been mistakes and dead ends along the way. There was excitement at something new discovered, followed by disappointment as I came to the edge of that way of understanding and realized that it did not go far enough, that I needed to go on searching.

For more than thirty-five years I have been working as a physician in palliative care. The emphasis in palliative care is on improving the quality of life of individuals living with serious illness through pain and symptom control and social, psychological, and spiritual support. Every day, I meet with people such as Ben and try to ease their pain and suffering so they can get on with living the fullest life possible. It gives me great joy when someone I am caring for finds healing, by which I mean freedom from suffering, a sense of aliveness, and peace of heart, even though she or he may be incurably ill or dying.

I am very grateful to be working as a doctor.

However, I have not always felt this way. My professional

journey began with a lot of ambivalence. Despite coming from a family steeped in the profession of medicine (my father, all four of my uncles, and both my grandfathers were doctors), I was not passionate about studying medicine, and there was never any pressure from my parents for me to become a doctor. One day, halfway through my studies, I was given a questionnaire to complete as part of a sociology research project aimed at determining why we students had chosen to study medicine. None of the suggested options rang true for me. The question that came closest was, "Are you studying medicine because you want to help people?" While I could check the "yes" box here, I knew that there was more to it than that. The science and technology of medicine did not excite me as it did many of my classmates. In addition, I felt dismayed by some of the care, or more accurately, the lack of care, that I saw being offered patients in the wards of our teaching hospital, especially to those with a terminal diagnosis.

I remember meeting Jack, a seventy-year-old man, during my first weeks on the wards. He was blind and had just been diagnosed with inoperable gastric cancer. His surgeon had "opened him up" a few days before but had not been able to do anything, and so he had just sewn his belly up again.

Jack was waiting to get news from the surgeon on his morning rounds about how the operation had gone. I had seen Jack on the day of his admission and got to know him on my daily visits since then. He was a wise, kind, and gentle soul.

I was anxious about how the meeting would go as the surgeon swept into the double room where Jack was, followed by a group of us junior medical students. The entourage stopped at the end of the other patient's bed while the surgeon spoke to him. As the surgeon talked, I was looking across at Jack and could see that he was sitting up alertly in bed, his dark glasses on, listening intently to the conversation with his roommate.

The surgeon finished talking to Jack's neighbor. But then, with the briefest of glances in Jack's direction, he turned around and left the room. The other students scuttled out of the room in the surgeon's wake. I just stood there looking at Jack, who seemed to be staring straight at me with an expression of incomprehension on his face. I felt a mixture of outrage at Jack's dismissive treatment and shame that I had not spoken up on his behalf. If this was what clinical medicine looked like, I did not want to be part of it.

During my years at medical school I lived with my parents in a house called Templehill on the banks of the River Lee, which neighbored a small cattle farm on the outskirts of Cork City in Ireland. I remember how happy I felt each day when my studies ended. Something in me seemed to open up when it was time to leave the alienation of the hospital and the city behind, and head for home.

As soon as I got there, I would collect my dog Bilbo, a small liver-brown and white English springer spaniel, and together we would head down to the river or up into the hills behind our house. I used to fish for salmon in the river. At weekends I hunted for pheasant, woodcock, and snipe with my Uncle Dick. I realized later that what I loved most about these hunting trips was having this time with my uncle and his dogs, and the long hours of walking in wild country and sitting silently at lakesides—watching and waiting. One day, Bilbo retrieved a wood pigeon I had shot, which was still alive but badly wounded and bleeding. As I took it from his mouth, it was still breathing. I felt its warm blood on my hand. I broke its neck to put it out of its misery and never hunted again.

I have always loved to be in nature. I find that in nature I can be undefended, I can be myself, and know a kind of peace and joy on which I can rely. When, on a Native American vision quest ceremony a couple of years ago, I was left alone on a mountainside in the wilderness to begin four days of fasting and praying, my strongest feelings were not of trepidation but of relief. As I lay down on the Earth, memories came flooding back of lying among the rushes at the side of the River Lee; the air full of the warming sun and the sounds of water flowing in the shallows. Then, as now, I felt happy and at peace.

As a child, I played outside a lot, either alone or with my brothers and friends. Every summer when I was young, I used to vacation with my family for three long months in Youghal, on the coast south of Cork. I spent each day outdoors with a gang of friends. We went to the beach to explore rock pools, catch shrimp and little fish called "cobblers," or just laze about with the stray dogs in the sunny grass by the railway tracks behind my grandparents' house. As a teenager, I liked to make Super 8 movies. I remember one I made about our wild and magnificent garden on the banks of the river at Templehill with images of swans, and sunsets, and the light reflecting on the river.

Then something happened that changed my relationship with nature. Two young women, friends of our family, drowned when a canoe they were in flipped over in the swimming hole right in front of our house, despite the valiant efforts of my then ten-year-old brother who had dived in to try to save them. In the weeks and months afterward, I began to realize that some sort of naiveté had died in me that day in the dark waters of the river. I could no longer simply look at nature as a beautiful refuge that was there for me when I needed her. Nature existed in her own right and on her own terms. Nature was also awful, ruthless, and mysterious. Yes, there was beauty in nature, great beauty, but there was also pain, separation, and death. Nature had a life of her own.

This marked the end of my idealized relationship with nature. Up until then what I loved about the natural world was its innocence. My favorite poets at school had been the English romantics. I remember turning to William Wordsworth again around this time, hoping to find words that would restore my primal garden. Instead, I found him talking about "something that is gone," in his relationship with the natural world, and asking, "Where is it now, the glory and the dream?"[2] Having my feelings and questions mirrored back to me like this brought me unexpected consolation. I realized that I was not alone in what I was feeling. It was as though I were standing barefoot on the earth.

At the beginning of my fourth year in medical school I had an encounter on the wards of the teaching hospital that prompted me to seriously consider leaving medicine. My mother had asked me to look in on her friend Jane, a woman in her fifties, who was dying with widespread breast cancer. She was a patient on the surgical ward where I was working as a medical student. I started visiting Jane regularly and began to get to know this quiet and lovely woman. One day when I arrived, I found her in a lot of pain. I went to speak with the nurse in charge, who told me that while medicines to relieve pain were available, she did not want to give them to Jane at this point, "In case she really needs them at the end."

As it turned out, the end was just a few weeks away and, sadly, Jane remained in pain for most of that time. While she did have some moments of respite, these had little if anything to do with her medical care. Jane loved classical music. She had suggested I buy a book about the appreciation of music that introduced different composers and their work and linked them to the visual art of the French Impressionists. Sometimes, after discussing a composer and looking at the images in the book together, we would listen to one of her favorite pieces on her CD player. At these times, she would close her eyes and, with a brief softening in how she held herself, for a little while sink more deeply into her pillows.

Even though I felt awkward and inadequate every time I entered her room, Jane always seemed pleased to see me and would thank me for my visit in a way that made me feel that she really meant it. I would leave her room with a sense that I too had received something from her. It was as though being present to each other in this way, despite our powerlessness to change anything about of her illness or her pain, had brought us both into a mutuality of comfort and consolation. But I was also frustrated and at times outraged to witness her awful, continuing physical pain. Was this the best that modern medicine, with all its technological prowess, could offer? There had to be a better way.

In 1974, during a spiritual retreat at University College Dublin, I met Jean Vanier, the Canadian Catholic philosopher and founder of L'Arche communities for people with developmental disabilities.[3] I told him that I was unhappy and disillusioned in my medical studies and thinking of leaving. He listened intently to all I had to say. When I finished, he said,

"Before you do, I suggest you visit a place in London called St Christopher's Hospice...." And then he added, "It's a place of healing."

I took Jean Vanier's advice. A few months later I attended a one-week multidisciplinary training course at St Christopher's. While there, I met patients who, though weak and frail, were some of the most complete human beings I have ever encountered. It was as though the fire of their illness had burnt away the nonessential and all that remained was their original selves.

I began to think more about what is meant by "healing." Clearly it was distinct from curing, in the sense of fixing or making better, if it was what I was witnessing here in these individuals so close to death. Suddenly I flashed back to the peaceful give and take of consolation that I had experienced with Jane. I knew at that moment I had discovered the answer to the question as to why I was studying medicine. Even if I had not fully understood what it meant at the time, I was being called to become a healer. I felt deeply encouraged by this insight and was able to return to Ireland and finish my studies.

In August 1980, I began working in St Christopher's and saw that in fact no one needed to suffer the way Jane had. With careful diagnosis and treatment, pain and other distressing symptoms could be relieved. I also learned that a healing environment could, in itself, have a powerful therapeutic effect. I was told that when I admitted a new patient in pain,

I should try not to make too many alterations or dose changes in medications during the first twenty-four hours because, for many, just being in this hospice environment and experiencing close attention and compassionate care for even a short period of time could have powerful therapeutic benefits.

Even though I was skeptical at first about this, I was surprised by a change I witnessed in a man called John. I remember this fifty-year-old man well as he was one of the first patients I admitted to St Christopher's. On admission the previous evening, he had been in severe pain from the lung cancer that had spread to his bones. He was already on a good regime of pain-relieving medications. I explained to him that I would not change anything that evening, that he could ask for extra pain medication as needed overnight, and that we would reassess and make whatever changes were needed when we saw him the next day.

The following morning, I found John sitting up in bed, looking relaxed and eating a piece of toast. When I asked him how he was doing, he replied, "I got some sleep last night. The pain is not so bad this morning." It seemed that something had shifted overnight and that this had nothing to do with any clever medical interventions. When John added, "For the first time in months, I'm feeling safe again," I began to understand that the change I was witnessing had something to do with a lessening of his fear. Suddenly I could see what Cicely Saunders, pioneer of the hospice movement, meant when she spoke of "total pain": that pain is not so much a self-contained entity as a multidimensional and dynamic process involving every aspect of an individual's experience, which is exacerbated by isolation and eased by coming back into relationship and community.[4]

I had just completed my first three months at St Christopher's when I had an experience that was to turn my world inside out. At that time, I was happy in my work. I looked forward to going into the hospice every day and was giving my patients and their families my all. While there were obvious limits to what I could offer in terms of my clinical and communication skills, I tried to make up for this by being as openhearted as possible. Day after day, I was in the presence of pain and grief on a scale I had not previously encountered. I thought that good intention, careful listening, and my newly acquired skills in treating pain and other symptoms were all I needed. As I sat with a patient, I would take it all in—their pain, their fear, their regrets, their grief, their sadness—and respond in whatever ways I could.

Unbeknownst to me, I was paying a psychological toll by absorbing such a relentless flow of human suffering. The very openness I was offering my patients was also making me vulnerable to their pain. Walking home each evening from the hospice to the apartment where I was living with my wife and our baby daughter, I felt simultaneously enriched and emotionally depleted.

The straw that broke the camel's back was a heartbreaking situation in which I had to tell three very young children that their mother was dying. As the patient's husband and the children left the room where a social worker and I had been meeting with them, I knew that what I had just said—that their mother would never be coming home again—had caused them unimaginable pain. In just a few words I had told them something that would change their lives. It was not necessarily that I had done it badly; there was no easy way to put it. When they filed out of the room silently ahead of their father, I did not move. I continued to sit there, feeling hollow.

The following day I came to work in a fog. A sensation of being mentally clouded lingered throughout the day and I noticed that I could not easily concentrate. I was aware of a sense of dread in my chest and I became more and more apprehensive. As I walked down the corridor, my heart was pounding and my mouth was dry. I bumped into the medical director, Tom West, and asked if I could speak with him. We went to his office.

Tom listened carefully as I told him what was happening. "You sound exhausted," he said. "I can see you're doing a great job, but I think you may not yet have learned that you also need to take care of yourself. Two suggestions. First, take this

Friday off. Make it a long weekend and think about going away somewhere nice with your family. Secondly, it might be helpful for you to have someone to meet with to talk to from time to time. I have been doing this for years and I would not have survived in this work without it."

My head was still reeling, but I felt relieved and grateful that Tom did not think that I was crazy to be feeling this way.

Early the following week I met with a therapist. In the weeks and months that followed, I began to understand that I had suffered psychological trauma as an infant that had made me especially vulnerable to situations such as the one I had encountered with the young children and their dying mother. When I was three months old, my own mother had become seriously ill with tuberculosis while travelling abroad. On returning home, she had been hospitalized for nine months and was considered lucky to survive. During this time she was quarantined and I was not allowed to see her. I am told that when I was led into her room after all that time apart, I had stood at the doorway looking in at her with wide eyes, not recognizing who she was.

The work I did with that therapist was the start of a journey of descent into the unconscious that I have been on ever since. While continuing in therapy, I studied and trained in the use of guided imagery, active imagination, and dreamwork. Initially I saw these activities as exclusively personal pursuits that ran in parallel to the rest of my life. However, as my studies led me further into the field of depth psychology and the work of Carl Jung, this changed. From reading Jung, I began to understand that the unconscious is more than a personal process. Jung describes those aspects of the unconscious beyond the personal as "the collective unconscious," and in his later work, comes to see this as a shared field of energy and information; something we as individuals participate in rather than possess. He writes, "The collective unconscious surrounds us on all sides…. It is more like an atmosphere in which we live than something that is found in us…. Also, it does not by any means behave merely psychologically; in the cases of so-called synchronicity it proves to be a universal substrate present in the environment rather than a psychological premise."[5] This way of thinking offered a bridge between the "inner work" I was doing on myself and the rest of my life in the world.

Through my studies of Jung, I was led to the mythological roots of Western health care. I learned about Chiron, the centaur—half man and half horse. One day, Chiron was wounded in the leg by a poisoned arrow, leaving him with a painful, gaping wound that would not heal. Supported on the shoulder of his daughter, Chiron wandered the meadows of the mountainside where he lived, looking for healing herbs. Even though these did not work for him, he became wise in their use. The sick and dying came to see him from far and wide in search of healing. Sometimes his herbal treatments cured their illnesses and sometimes not. However, even if they were not cured, each one who encountered Chiron left feeling understood. In being attended to by someone who was also suffering, they felt more whole. They called Chiron "the wounded healer."

That title rang true. It described something that had not been named in my medical studies but that resonated for me in my work. I was fascinated to learn that at the roots of Western medicine was a figure who embodied a fusion of human and other-than-human nature.

Chiron was mentor to many of the great Greek mythological heroes. One of these was Asklepios, who had been brought to Chiron as an orphan. Asklepios became Chiron's favorite pupil. Chiron adopted him as a son and taught him all that he knew about the healing arts. Asklepios became a great healer, and was later immortalized as the Greek god of healing. For over a thousand years, pilgrims journeyed for healing to temples dedicated to Asklepios and his daughter Hygieia throughout the mainland and islands of Greece.

What happened at these temples was a healing ritual called

"dream incubation." Here the patient slept on the ground of the temple for the night and welcomed whatever came, dream or vision, as an epiphany, a visit from the god or goddess of healing. The practice honored the patient's potential for self-healing that could be awakened in the right circumstances. As mythologist Carl Kerényi puts it, "The physician cannot act alone; side by side with his outside intervention, something inside the patient must lend a helping hand if a cure is to be accomplished. At the crucial moment, something is at work that might best be compared to the flow of a spring."[6]

I was excited to learn that nature has been at the heart of healing from the beginnings of Western medicine. The temples of Asklepios were situated in surroundings of great natural beauty close to springs of flowing water. When someone arrived at a healing temple, she began a process of preparation and purification. When the time was right, the "incubant" was led at dusk to the temple. After making some ritual offerings, the priests would invite her to lie down on the ground. Everything led up to this moment. Lying down on the earth in the utter abandonment of sleep was the final and crucial step in doing all that could be done to enable healing to happen. The next move was not up to the physicians, or the priests, or the incubant herself. Healing, if and when it happened, came literally from the ground up, as the earth was seen as the origin of dreams.

I have a photograph I took of the healing temple at Lissos on the island of Crete. Situated in a wild and beautiful landscape, its sandstone walls line a mosaic floor that has been worn through by the feet of countless pilgrims since the third century BCE. The open, empty space of the temple speaks to me of what I can and cannot do to help another come into an experience of healing. While I cannot make someone experience healing in the way I can control their pain, for example, there is much I can do to create the environment and circumstances that make it more likely that this will happen. The landscape around the temple, the towering sandstone cliffs behind it, the giant, ancient olive trees close by, remind me how nature is at the very heart of the healing process. There is a spring there that runs to this day, the same fountain from which the incubants would have drunk. The day I visited, someone who had been there just before me told me that he had seen a snake—the symbol of Asklepios and of healing in the ancient world.

I realized why I was so at odds with the study and practice of Western medicine: it had forgotten its origins in the myths of Chiron and Asklepios and the principle they represent of working with nature for the healing of suffering. Instead, Western medicine had invested its all in the historical figure of Hippocrates and his method of deductive reasoning and evidence-based biological materialism. The key operating principle of the Hippocratic method is summarized in the phrase *opus contra naturam*,[7] "working against nature." While I could see clearly how we sometimes need anti-biotics, and anti-inflammatories, and anti-cancer drugs, it also seemed to me that beyond this literalism, there was anthropomorphic arrogance and a profound disrespect for the healing power of nature.

In the early 1990s, while working with the palliative care team at St Vincent's Hospital in Dublin, I met James, who had an inoperable tumor of his esophagus. This had shown up as an incidental finding when he was admitted with a heart attack, which he barely survived. His doctors had not told him about the cancer because they were concerned that he might not be able to cope with any more bad news. We had been consulted to see him for palliative care because he was desperately short of breath and very anxious. On the Friday afternoon when I first met him, he was so breathless that he was hardly able to talk. I recommended some changes to his medications to help his symptoms and promised to come back to see him after the weekend.

When I walked into James's ward the following Monday afternoon and greeted him, I was surprised when he sat up in bed and greeted me in return. I asked him how he was feeling. He replied, "Last night I had the most amazing dream of my life." I asked him to tell me about it. As he began to talk, his face lit up and his words flowed. He told me that in his dream a man had come to his bedside and woken him, and then taken him to the subterranean, Neolithic burial chamber of Newgrange in County Meath. This man had led James through a tunnel to the center of the tomb, and asked him to lean back against the tombstone. He then told him to walk out again. He gave James a shovel and told him to "start digging." As James did so he discovered that buried beneath Newgrange was another "pre-ancient" city. As James saw the circular walls of the houses and the straight lines of stones that marked the side of a road, he knew that he had unearthed something of great value. He looked straight at me and said, "It was as if I had discovered gold!"

James finished by saying; "I was frightened before I had that dream. I'm not frightened anymore." In the days that followed, he continued to weaken and never made it home as he had hoped. Despite not talking openly about dying, he quietly took care of his business. His wife and three sons were at his bedside when he gently slipped away.

What I learned from listening to James is that in working with dreams and the imagination in fluid and spontaneous ways, we are working with nature—our "inner nature." I came to see that much of our suffering comes from disconnection from our own deepest nature, and that this inevitably gives rise to feelings of isolation, alienation, and meaningless. I learned that sometimes a person's symptoms, be they physical, such as James' shortness of breath, or psychological, such as his fear, have an underlying deeper diagnosis of disconnection from our deepest selves, and that simply offering respect and hospitality to our dreams enables us to tap into a wisdom that is not just personal but shared, universal, and Earth-based. This inner nature connection practice can ease our suffering by offering us an accessible path out of isolation and back into relationship.

I also saw what happened for James as a move from head to heart. By "heart" I am not simply referring to what Brian Doyle calls "the wet engine" that pumps us through our lives.[8] I mean the heart as the source of wisdom and compassion; the heart as hub in a cosmic web of connectedness, where countless invisible threads radiate out in all directions. I saw that those who were the least afraid, and seemed to have the easiest times in their dying, were those who had come into their heart's estate.

At the bedside, helping my patients die with peace of heart involves doing all that I can, day after day, to alleviate their pain and suffering. But it's not just about how skilled I am at what I do. It's as much about *how* I do what I do. It matters that I listen deeply to my patients, that I act with kindness, and that I am able to wait, knowing that it's not all up to me, trusting that my patients carry within themselves an innate capacity for healing. When I act in this way, with close attention and care and, above all, with humility, I notice that it lessens both my own and my patient's anxiety, creates security, and opens up a space where healing may happen. And when this occurs, as it did for James, I am every time as surprised and delighted as my patient is. I know that the patient and I are in the presence of a process that is beyond our intelligence that has its own agency. I appreciate why my Native American teachers speak of this as the work of "The Great Mystery."

Through the 1990s and into the early years of this millennium, in my own search for healing, I experienced a growing desire to be closer to the natural world. I sought out the work of those who talked about the Earth as animate and intimate, including Irish writer John Moriarty and American writers Barry Lopez, Gary Snyder, and Mary Oliver. I came across the story of the Lakota Holy Man, Nicholas Black Elk. The book about his life coauthored with John Neihardt, *Black Elk Speaks*, ends with a poignant story that awoke in me what felt like a deep, forgotten grief.

This is the description of what happened when, as an old man, Black Elk returned to Harney Peak in the Black Hills of South Dakota and to the exact spot where, as a child, he had received a powerful vision of the healing of his people. As he stood there holding the sacred pipe and offering prayers to his ancestors, he began to weep. In words of despair he talked about how he believed he had failed in helping to realize what his vision had foretold. John Neihardt, who was with him on that occasion, ends the book with these words:

> We who listened now noted that thin clouds had
> gathered about us. A scant chill rain began to fall and
> there was low, muttering thunder without lightning.
> With tears running down his cheeks, the old man
> raised his voice to a thin high wail, and chanted, 'In
> sorrow I am sending a feeble voice, O Six Powers of
> the World. Hear me in my sorrow, for I may never call
> again. O make my people live!' For some minutes the
> old man stood silent, with face upturned, weeping in
> the drizzling rain. In a little while the sky was clear
> again.[9]

In October 2005, I was sitting in a coffee shop after work
with my friend Mario. I had told him the story of Black Elk,
and how moved I was by it. I had shared with him how I would
love to learn more about Native American ways of seeing and
being in the world. Mario told me about a Native American
community he had been introduced to by his Buddhist teacher,
Shinzen Young, which welcomed anyone who was interested in
this way of prayer. He invited me to come with him to a sweat
lodge ceremony he was planning to attend at their mountain
camp the following weekend.

I was both excited and anxious at the prospect. I also had concerns about coming to an Native American ceremony as a white man and a European, one whose ancestors had done so much damage to Native North American peoples by stealing their lands, killing the animals they depended on, and destroying their way of life. From 1884, when the United States formally outlawed "pagan" ceremonies, until the American Indian Religious Freedom Act in 1978, it was illegal for the Indian people of North America to practice some aspects of their religious rituals; during that time someone who was caught leading or participating in a ceremony such as the one I was about to attend could have been imprisoned. I was aware that to this day some Indians did not want non-Native people to participate in their ceremonies, being justifiably wary and suspicious of their motives.

The following Saturday, Mario and I drove along in silence through the harsh beauty of the high desert. On our arrival, he introduced me to Wolf and Lisa Wahpepah, the leaders of the intertribal spirit camp and keepers of lifelong vows to preserve their Native traditions. They welcomed me warmly, and I joined some other newcomers in a circle in the shade of an old white pine close to the fireplace.

Wolf began, "When we crawl into the lodge, we say *'For all my relations!'* When we Indians say, *'All my relations,'* we're not just referring to our blood relatives or even all other humans; we're talking about all living beings on Mother Earth, including the plants, and the rocks, and the waters, as well as Grandmother moon, and Grandfather Sun, and all the celestial bodies."

From then on, I have continued to pray with this fireplace and all who gather there, and I regularly participate in their ceremonies. The fierce and beautiful container that is the sweat lodge ceremony has become a safe place to bring my personal pain and the residues of pain I am carrying in my heart for my patients. I go there to grieve, and to express gratitude, and to pray. On more than one occasion, I have spent time "up on the hill" on vision quest, which has been an opportunity to lie on the earth with my questions and my not knowing, to stay there long enough for the earth's rhythm to become my rhythm. As a Celt, something in my soul feels deeply at home on the Red Road of Native American spirituality. Through these elemental ways of prayer, I have come into a deeper relationship with the land and with nature. The worldview that is "All my relations" now permeates my work in palliative care and my relationships with others and the world.

At the same time, I was also becoming familiar with the work of Buddhist scholar, deep ecologist, and activist Joanna Macy. Radhule had brought Joanna's book, *Mutual Causality in Buddhism and General Systems Theory*, home with her from a retreat she had attended and it became our shared bedtime reading. In the book Joanna explores the core insight in the enlightenment of Siddhartha Gautama, the historical Buddha: what in Pali is called *paticca samuppada*, meaning "mutual causality" or "dependent co-arising." She explains that in contrast to our usual ways of understanding causality as a linear process between discrete, solid objects (like billiard balls hitting one another), *paticca samuppada* implies that what manifests as reality is, in fact, a dynamic, fluid, interconnected, and interdependent process, where "everything arises through mutual conditioning in reciprocal interaction."[10]

Radhule had also introduced me to the guided meditations of Buddhist scholar and teacher Alan Wallace some years earlier, and mindfulness of breathing had become an important daily practice for me. I found one detail in Alan's instructions especially helpful: he asks the meditator to bring particular attention to the exhalation of the breath, and then to, "Release and let go all the way through the exhale and continue to let go even beyond the end of the exhale until the next breath flows in effortlessly, like a wave washing up on shore."[11] Following this guidance to continue in the trajectory of letting go beyond the end of the exhale, something very simple yet profound happens: I discover that the body breathes all by itself, without my having to do anything! This may seem to be stating the obvious, but by consciously noticing my breath and allowing myself to align with it, I find that I am being carried in the effortless flow of the body's natural rhythms.

As I engaged in this practice daily, I noticed that something unexpected was happening. I was learning to trust the body's natural autonomy. Allowing the body to breathe like this brought me, at times, to what Sufi mystic Kabir describes as, "The place [inside me] where the world is breathing."[12] From here, every morning, I would walk with our dogs onto the land behind our house. Arriving in the landscape in this way, with a quiet mind, I could vividly sense the light, the birdsong, the coolness of the air on my cheek, the smell of the damp earth. And when I stopped close to where an unseen bird was singing in a tree, and closed my eyes and listened, I realized that I was not just listening with my ears; my whole body was receptive and registering the vibrations of sound.

Up until then, I had a prejudice that Buddhist teachings were dualistic, valuing awareness and detachment over matter and engagement. That is why I was so excited to learn about *paticca samuppada* and "engaged Buddhism," from Joanna. Here were Buddhist teachings that did not encourage disassociation or separation from the world. Rather, they showed that we are inextricably linked to our world; indeed, that we are the world.

For over thirty years Joanna Macy has been offering seminars and workshops inspired by the teaching of the radical interdependence of all life, which offer practices to enable us to move from passivity to action on behalf of our suffering world.[13] I was struck by how congruent this Buddhist science of mind and heart and the new science of systems thinking are with the indigenous teaching that "all are relatives."

In the late fall of 2012, I attended one of Joanna's Work That Reconnects workshops. At the introductory session on the first evening, person after person spoke of their pain and anger, their frustration and despair because of what was happening to our planet. Climate scientist Susanne Moser told us that grief-work is the most relevant emotional work we can do, and spoke of "hospice care for our dying planet." Nuclear scientists Kathleen Sullivan and Arnie Gundersen talked to us about the ongoing implications of the nuclear meltdown at Fukushima. And artist Chris Jordan spoke of a movie he was making about the albatrosses on Midway Island, as he shared images of dead baby birds, their stomachs ruptured by shards of plastic their parents had skimmed from the surface of the Pacific while hunting for food and unwittingly fed to them.

I was troubled by the dawning awareness of what all this meant for my children, and their children, and for all the grandchildren of our world. Just before I had left for the workshop, my eldest daughter had called to tell me that she was pregnant. As I listened now, some spoke of how we may already have passed a point of no return with climate change, that it may already be too late to prevent the sort of consequences that will make it difficult for complex life forms to survive. A young couple shared their decision not to bring children into such an ailing and uncertain world. What, I asked myself, did all this mean for my little grandchild to be, who, all going well, would take her or his first breath in this world in just a few short months? At that moment, it was as though something within me crumbled and fell to the ground. I remember feeling shocked, exposed, and raw.

In July 2013, I held my newborn first-grandchild, Elliot, in my arms. As I looked at his tiny sleeping body, I wondered what the world would be like in sixty years' time, when he was my age. I realized that if even a fraction of the predictions I was hearing of environmental, economic, and cultural collapse came true, he would be living in a different and a very much more difficult world.

Whereas before I had dealt with things that happened to the environment with a certain distance and lack of feeling, I found that this was no longer an option. My growing closer to other-than-human nature had sensitized me to its welfare; the birth of my grandchild made *everything* personal. I was gutted when I saw that the new owners of our previous home had pulled up all the plants I had tended there over the years, including the great white sage whose cuttings I used to bring to the sweat lodge as gifts for Wolf and Lisa. I was shocked and then saddened the day I walked down the road with the dogs and saw that the owners of the new house by the corner had cut down two of their three big ash trees, where flocks of robins used to gather in the Fall. And I was sickened when I read about the beautiful three-year-old female wolf called Echo who had travelled all the way from Wyoming to the brink of the Grand Canyon in Utah only to be killed by a hunter's bullet. Would Elliot grow up in a world where there were no wolves left in the wild?

As I opened to the pain of the world in this way, I felt at times overwhelmed by a tsunami of suffering. My old self would have liked to block this out, but I realized that denial was no longer an option. I noticed that I was deliberately trying to numb myself by overworking, or by overworrying, or by distracting myself in various ways, but that this, at best, bought temporary relief. I was at a loss. While I had become an expert in managing pain in my professional life, I had no idea what to do with the pain I was now feeling.

RELATING TO PAIN

For as long as I can remember, I have dreaded pain (by which I mean what I experience as distressing and uncomfortable) and done all that I could to avoid it. As the eldest of six boys with one older sister, I tried my hardest to keep things calm and make things better in what I experienced as a mostly loving but at times turbulent home. My father was a surgeon who often drank heavily when he came home in the evenings, leading to arguments between him and my mother. Not infrequently this ended with my mother slamming the door and running out of the house in tears, driving off into the night. It hurt me to see my mother so upset and I tried as hard as I could to make her happy. I became the peacemaker, to the best of my ability, between my parents. I used to sit between them at the dinner table and attempt to mediate a truce when things were tense by leading the conversation in what I thought would be a safe direction.

If this did not work, as it often did not, I would take Bilbo and together we would climb the hill behind our house, where we would walk for hours through fields of corn stubble and little wooded areas, listening to the call of the cock pheasant, or the snipe that Bilbo had flushed from the marshy reed beds. At the top of the hill there was just the wind, more hills as far as I could see to the west, and the meandering silver sash of river. Planes, lights on now as dusk darkened, circled on their approach to Cork Airport. Slowly, imperceptibly, my fluttering heart would drop into a slower, deeper rhythm until eventually I had circled back to where our house was directly down below. There I would pause, and watch, as lights began to flicker on in the windows, and brace myself for my descent.

My fear of pain and my desire to avoid it was certainly a factor (even if an unconscious one) in how I ended up in a medical specialty where the primary focus is on pain and symptom management. Pain is controlled using the traditional medical model by firstly diagnosing its cause, and then treating it by means of evidence-based interventions. The medical model is effective and helpful to many much of the time. It can prevent and cure disease, ease pain and suffering, and improve the quality of life of patients living with chronic and terminal illnesses. It has been a good match for me with my pain phobia, affording me a protective barrier of clinical objectivity as I attend to my patients. What is more, the result of a successful therapeutic encounter is relief all round: a lessening of pain and anxiety—the patient's, and mine.

However, the medical model does not always work. It has little to offer Ben whose life is coming to an end too soon, and could not comfort those three little children when their mother was dying, as they looked back at me with an expression I could only begin to understand.

When I realized there was no way that I could give Ben

the reassurance that he would recover from his illness and get back to life as before, I felt powerless, inadequate, and guilty. I was physically uncomfortable. There was an edgy tension in my body that made it hard for me to stay in the room with him. I desperately wanted to open the door and go outside and get some air. From experience, I recognized these feelings and sensations for what they were: a by now familiar pattern of what happens when I hit the limits of what I can do to ease another's suffering. Seeing this for what it was helped. It afforded me a choice. I could either leave Ben's room, as every cell in my body was pleading with me to do ("Let me go and find our social worker to come and sit with you"), or I could, despite my discomfort, choose to stay with him, as one human being to another, hoping that this might bring him some deeper consolation, even if it was not the answer he was hoping for.

From my studies in depth psychology, I had learned that this way of being with another in suffering had a name: this was the path of the wounded healer, the path forged by Chiron. The path of the wounded healer can be summarized as follows: by staying with our woundedness, we encourage the other to stay with theirs; that is where and how healing happens. The wounded healer is one who knows that everyone carries within themselves an innate potential for healing. The wounded healer is one who knows from experience that, paradoxically, this potential within is realized by staying with what hurts. The wounded healer knows that waiting with our own suffering, while being present and empathic to the other, is what encourages the other to stay with theirs. The wounded healer agrees with Rumi when he says, "Don't turn your head. Keep looking at the bandaged place. That's where the light enters you."[1]

With the path of the wounded healer, I had found a second way of being with pain. In contrast to the medical model, which only worked when there was a "fixable" pain, the path of the wounded healer offered me another, positive way of being with one whose pain was "unfixable." I now had a powerful conceptual incentive to stay with patients like Ben with an open heart, waiting, and being present to him in his grief and his despair even when there was nothing left for me to do, hoping that this would help to transform his suffering. The core teaching of the wounded healer is that in suffering our suffering together, we come into the mystery of healing.

In 2008, I was invited to be lead author of an article on self-care for physicians working at the end of life for *The Journal of the American Medical Association* (*JAMA*).[2] This prompted a year of research and creative collaboration with four coauthors and gave me a deeper understanding of the dynamics of resilience. I learned about burnout, the emotional and physical depletion that results from organizational stress, a form of low-grade suffering that is endemic to caregivers. I learned about secondary traumatic stress disorder, also known as "compassion fatigue," when we are vicariously traumatized by another's suffering, and realized that this is what I had experienced all those years before when I first began working at St Christopher's Hospice.

It seemed clear to me and my coauthors that traditional models of self-care, which emphasized the importance of having "good professional boundaries" to protect ourselves from the stresses of the workplace, coupled with replenishing programs of rest and renewal outside the workplace for when we are off-duty, were only part of the solution. We argued that, in addition to these traditional models of self-care, we needed ways of practicing self-care that would both protect and replenish us *within* the workplace.

We proposed a model of self-care based on self-awareness. Here self-awareness, which we described as a combination of self-knowledge and mindfulness, is in itself protective, allowing us to self-monitor and consider how we are going to respond moment by moment in any given situation. It allows us to choose to step back or ask for help from other members of our team when we need to, and it allows us to move in closer to our patients when we want to. If our choice is to stay with the one who is suffering, our heartfelt presence opens a channel of connection, which lessens the intensity of the patient's distress and allows us both to emerge enriched by the encounter.

At the time I was writing the *JAMA* article, I had been in

the field of end-of-life care for almost thirty years. I was working full-time as a physician with hospital and community-based palliative care teams, and as medical director of an inpatient hospice in Santa Barbara, California. While I loved the people I was working with, I noticed that I was no longer excited, as I had been in those early years at St Christopher's, to go to work each morning. Instead, I was feeling emotionally and physically run down most of the time. I no longer had that inner "hum" that had been there in the past, which came from knowing that I was in my chosen profession and doing the right work. Even after a restful weekend, my energy was flat. More often than not, I felt unhappy with the quality of my work. I had the pervasive feeling that I was not doing what I really wanted to do and was doing too much of what I did not want to do, and I frequently found myself fantasizing about leaving medicine. I remember the moment I realized one evening, as I was reading a paper on the symptoms of burnout, that I was experiencing every symptom on the list: that I was burnt out.

I asked myself how this could have happened, given that I had been practicing both the traditional and self-awareness models of self-care I was promoting in the article. I had good boundaries around my work and I took vacations. I had been in therapy and clinical supervision for many years. I practiced mindfulness. I worked with my dreams. I exercised. I gardened. I did not smoke or drink. I was happy in my home life. Again and again, I returned to the thought that maybe I was no longer doing the right kind of work. Maybe the issue was that the river of my soul had turned and was moving in a new direction, leaving me high and dry in the rut of my old day job. Or was it that I underestimated the toll of organizational stress, the slow grinding down that comes with having to wrestle every day with the cold, gray bureaucracy of health care?

It was around this time that I took a scheduled summer vacation. I spent two weeks with my family in West Cork in Ireland. I had a wonderful time and returned to work rested and replenished. I remember my first morning back, walking into the inpatient palliative care office at 9:00 a.m. that Monday morning. One of my colleagues commented on how relaxed I looked. We chatted a little and then began the morning routine of going through our list of patients, triaging as we went who would see whom.

The nurse who had worked the weekend filled us in on each patient. The first person she talked about was Frank. Frank was fifty-three years old and had a long history of lung disease. He now had anoxic brain injury following a heart attack and cardiac arrest. He had been on a ventilator for several days and attempts to wean him off had so far been unsuccessful. He was a widower and caretaker of a young family, including a ten-year-old daughter with severe disability from cerebral palsy. He had no advance directive and was "Full Code" (meaning that everything possible would be done to resuscitate him in case of a cardiac or respiratory arrest). There was disagreement between the patient's children and his siblings about the future direction his care should take. A family meeting was scheduled for 10:00 a.m. Without pause, the nurse moved on to the next patient, a forty-two-year-old woman with advanced ovarian cancer who was suffering pain and vomiting due to bowel obstruction, and the next, a thirty-six-year-old man with a nonhealing compound fracture of his tibia and fibula with osteomyelitis, acute on chronic pain and opioid tolerance, and the next, a ninety-six-year-old woman who had had a massive stroke and shown no signs of improvement in almost a week but whose daughter wanted everything done, including placement of a tracheostomy and a feeding tube. These were just the first four patients; there were twelve more to go.

As I listened to this litany of human suffering, I felt like a soft-shelled crab. It was painful to hear these stories. I noticed that I was tightening up and pulling back to try to protect myself from what I was hearing. It was just too much. I found myself thinking that those of us who work with pain and suffering every day hugely underestimate the toll our psyches are taking. We focus on fixing what can be fixed and having the conversations that can be had; we negotiate the politics and the egos of the workplace; we do our best with the family dynamics; meanwhile, we have already started to engage with the next story of suffering, and the next, and the next. At that moment, I became aware of what felt like an old, aching hurt in the center of my chest. I saw that good boundaries, enjoyable times out, and even self-awareness practices were simply not enough. I remembered Dr. C., the medical oncologist we had interviewed for our *JAMA* article, who had said, "The stuff that burns me out has nothing to do with loss; it's fighting with insurance companies." And I realized that for me, in contrast to Dr. C., it was the opposite: it was precisely the accumulated losses and daily encounters with human pain and suffering that were burning me out.

Neither of the two ways of being with pain that I had learned so far, what I have called the medical model and the path of the wounded healer, were of much help to me here, in the face of such suffering. As I thought about this I slowly began to realize why. What I had learned so far had taught me a lot: from the medical model, I had learned how to diagnose and treat another's "fixable" pain, and, with the path of the wounded healer, I had found a potentially transformative way of being with another in their "unfixable" pain. However, what was totally missing was any real instruction on what to do with *my own pain*. I had not been taught about what to do with what I was experiencing in the face of another's anguish. I saw clearly that it was precisely this—not knowing what to do with the pain *I was experiencing*—that was leading to my feeling overwhelmed and burnt out. I knew that I had to find another way, a better way, of being with pain.

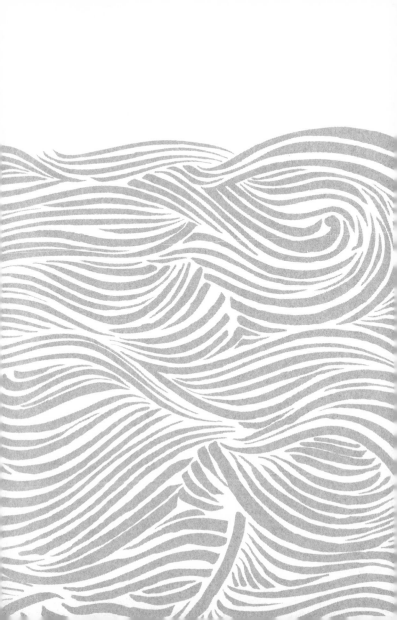

Seven Stories of Nature Connection

In my quest to find another way of being with pain, I want to share seven stories of encounters I had with other-than-human nature. While these stories are personal in a subjective and biographical sense, my hope is that the effect on the reader may be like time spent alone in the wilderness, or like sinking your hands deep into soft, dark earth and letting your fingers linger there for a while. Time spent in and with other-than-human nature, with an attitude of deep listening and respect, can reorganize us into someone closer to our original selves.

I share these stories in the spirit of the Buddha's teaching on the nature of suffering and the nature of healing, the Four Noble Truths. The First Noble Truth is the truth of suffering: *suffering exists.* I share these stories because we are suffering, and the Earth is suffering. The Second Noble Truth is the truth of the cause of suffering: *suffering has a cause.* I share these stories because suffering comes from our clinging to the delusion that we are separate from the rest of nature. The Third Noble Truth is the truth of the cessation of suffering: *healing is possible.* I share these stories because our suffering ceases when we know that we are inseparable from the rest of nature. And the Fourth Noble Truth is the truth of the path to the cessation of suffering: *there is a path to healing.*

I share these stories because connecting to other-than-human nature helps us to remember that we are seamless parts of the living whole, that we are all "relatives." Each story expresses how we can find healing through what Jon Young, tracker, author, and leader in the new nature movement, calls "deep nature connection."[1] Connection with other-than-human nature is a powerful medicine. I have experienced this personally through my experiences on the Red Road and in times I have spent in the natural world.

Nature connection, the process of connecting with other-than-human-nature through sensory awareness, is a deceptively simple yet extraordinary practice that can bring us insight and healing. As we connect with other-than-human-nature we realize that our world consists of countless other lives, each with their own uniqueness, and aliveness, and awareness, and that no single life is autonomous; each life exists only and because of its relationships of interdependence with others. Nature connection is about allowing this understanding to wash through us, helping us to remember that our deeper identity is one of what Zen

Buddhist teacher Thich Nhat Hahn calls "interbeing."[2]

I have seen how, when nature connection happens in even very small ways, it can bring us from isolation to relatedness, ease our pain, and improve the quality of our lives. The more deeply we experience our interconnectedness with the rest of nature, the more awake and alive we become, and the more we care about others and our world.

The stories that follow tell of how, through increasing immersion in the teachings of nature, I came upon a way of being with pain that I have found to be personally transformative. Here was a way of being with pain that enlivened and sustained rather than deadened and drained; a way of being with pain that awakened compassion and a yearning to ease the suffering and enable the healing of others.

FIRST

_____

COLMAN'S WELL

At the turn of the new millennium, my marriage of twenty-three years ended. As part of a turbulent and traumatic process for everyone involved and through circumstances not of my choosing, I did not get to see my three daughters, who at that time ranged in ages from sixteen to twenty-one, for over a year.

During these hardest of times there were moments of respite. My meditation practice helped, as did time in nature. Late at night I took long walks in a cold wind under the stars on Sandymount Strand in Dublin.

Later, back in my small, upstairs apartment, in what became a ritual of surrender, I would lie face down on a wolf robe (fur) in front of a small homemade altar of meaningful photos and artifacts, and find some respite in the softness and smell of the fur and the solidity of the floor. I found solace in the words from R. S. Thomas's poem "Here": "It is too late to start/ For destinations not of the heart. / I must stay here with my hurt."[1] At times, I found that I arrived at a deeper spaciousness, a peace of heart, and that I could breathe again. I missed my daughters intensely. I was reminded of the unrelenting pain of homesickness I had experienced during the six years I spent at boarding school. The school was in the west of Ireland, on rolling farmland dotted with lakes and old oak forests. I remembered how then, as now, I had wandered with an aching heart out on the land. I remembered how, then, as now, when I had sat and watched and waited, I had felt less alone.

It was late afternoon at the end of January 2000 as I approached the little forest over stony ground. I was careful about how I placed my feet on the limestone slabs that had been rounded by millennia of Atlantic rain and winds. When I came to the trees under the hillside, I knew that I had arrived.

There was the well; a horseshoe-shaped stone structure about as high as my chest, with water flowing into it at its base from the passing stream. Looking over the sidewall of the well, I saw that its soft muddy bottom was covered with crystal clear water a few inches deep. All around were trees and ferns and dappled light.

This well in the Burren in County Clare dates back one-and-a-half thousand years to an early Irish monastic settlement founded by Colman Mac Duagh, a bishop in the early Irish church. It is still a place of pilgrimage for many who came there to pray. Pilgrims leave token offerings of little pieces of brightly colored cloth hanging in the branches of the willows growing over the well.

On this particular day, I was aching and confused, feeling severed from my daughters. I had come here because I knew it as a refuge, a sacred place, a place of beauty. I had come because I knew there would be no judgment here, and no explanations needed. Here was a place where I could be my undefended self.

I found a flat, dry patch of ground alongside the stream, close to the opening of the well, and lay down. I was physically and emotionally exhausted. I closed my eyes. My body felt like lead. I collapsed onto the cold, firmness of the rock. Lying there I could hear the trickle of the water flowing over stones just inches away. There was birdsong, and the brushing of the leaves of the willows overhead. I could picture their branches, arched and sweeping back and forth. Even though all was dark, there were flashes of gold as spots of sunlight touched my face. And all the while there was the hungry, ragged aching in the center of my chest.

I don't know how long I had been asleep when I was awakened by an unusual sound nearby. For some time, I continued to lie there without moving, listening with my eyes closed to what seemed to be a scratching noise. When I opened my eyes, I saw a robin, with his small brown body and russet breast. He was directly in front of me, maybe three feet away, at the edge of the stream. He continued to scratch the ground, flipping over stones, hunting for insects. He stopped. He was even closer to me now. I was still lying there on my side, facing him. He raised his head, tilted it slightly, and looked right at me. I found myself looking into the tiny black pool of the robin's eye. For maybe two or three seconds he held my gaze; then he turned away and went back to hunting and feeding.

I watched the robin as he continued his winding journey downstream and out of sight. Then I turned over, lay on my back and looked up. I could see patches of blue sky through the green canopy of the overhead trees. I noticed that something had changed in how I was feeling that was difficult to put my finger on. It was as though my heart had come into a steadier beat. Or that something had opened in me that felt like remembering, or being remembered.

With this an image came. I saw my three girls. They were

here too, but they were not alone. My eldest daughter, Mary-Anna, was with my grandfather George, sitting, as a younger version of herself, on his knee, as if he were telling her a story. My middle daughter, Claire, was with my mother, Anne, both standing side by side, smiling and looking alike. My youngest daughter Ruth was with my grandmother Delia, who had her arms around her. I was still aware of the aching but it was different now. Its edges were softer and it seemed to be reaching out to the rocks and the trees rather than pulling back into itself.

When I was preparing to leave the well, I could not find my glasses. I had laid my new, very expensive glasses on the ground when I lay down. Now they were gone and, despite thirty minutes of searching, they were nowhere to be found. As I walked in a blur across the limestone paving back to where my car was parked, Rainer Maria Rilke's words came to mind: "The work of the eyes is done. Go now and do the heart work ..."[2]

SECOND

THE OTHER SIDE OF THE ROAD

In November 2007, I was in Gardiner, Montana, adjacent to the northern entrance of Yellowstone National Park. I had been fascinated by wolves for some time and was following their reintroduction into Yellowstone with avid interest. Up until then I had only ever seen them in captivity. I wanted to see a wolf in the wild and had arranged to spend a day in the park with a wolf biologist. We did see some wolves that day but only as small specks through binoculars, and, although we did have encounters with bison, elk, coyotes, mountain sheep, and a golden eagle, I was disappointed as I returned to my motel room. Later that evening I went back into the park alone.

I decided to go to the west side of Yellowstone to visit an information center there before it closed. As I drove along, I passed large herds of elk on the land to either side of the road. A car approached me, flashing its lights. I realized I was driving too fast and slowed down. Another car approached, also flashing its lights. I understood then that the drivers were warning me about something up ahead, so I slowed down even more. As I turned the next corner, I saw what appeared to be a large gray dog approaching on my side of the road. I pulled my car into the curb on the opposite side and slowed to a halt maybe fifty yards ahead of what I now realized was an approaching wolf.

The wolf continued to come toward me, staying by the tree line at the side of the road. He was going where he was going and he did not seem too bothered by my presence. As he passed me, his gait was graceful and effortless. His mouth was slightly open and he was looking straight ahead.

I understood that as a visitor to Yellowstone, I should keep my distance from wild animals, and that it could be dangerous, even lethal, not to do so. However, as I watched the wolf walk away in my rearview mirror, I knew I had to follow. I turned my car around and drove along slowly some twenty or thirty yards behind the wolf. He stayed on the left-hand curb and continued at the same pace. For some time we traveled along like this.

As we turned a corner, I saw a car fast approaching but still some ways off. I accelerated, overtook the wolf, and flashed my headlights to signal to the driver to slow down. He did, and pulled into the curb to let the wolf pass. I too pulled into the curb ahead of the wolf and waited and watched in my rearview mirror as he approached. When he passed he did not look in my direction and never changed his pace. I was aware that my heart was beating fast, yet I felt calm.

I restarted the car and continued to follow the wolf. Then, suddenly, he turned, crossed over a small, wooden footbridge to his left, and disappeared into the pines. I pulled my car into the curb and turned off the engine. I sat back in my seat and closed my eyes. I was stunned. I was wide awake.

That night, I felt so excited that I had trouble getting to sleep. I don't remember what I dreamt about but I do remember waking up with the desire to recall every detail of my meeting with the wolf. I had a feeling in my chest that was hard to define. It felt like a mix of hunger-pain and homesickness. As I lay on my bed thinking about what had happened, I realized that what

I was feeling was a longing to be close to the wolf. I wanted to see him again. I wanted to cross the road to be with him.

Since then, from time to time, I flash back to the meeting with the wolf. I see his face, his partially open mouth, his hint of a smile, his utter self-possession, and the liquidity of his movements—so that he is not so much walking, or running, as flowing. I see the blackness of the road, its miles of asphalt, and the unfathomable distance between us. And more and more frequently now I see that little bridge that led from the road to the firs and the new snow on the brown grass beyond. I see him crossing over, and disappearing behind the firs. I see the empty bridge now, standing there. And I am standing there too, filled with longing.

What, I have asked myself, over and over since then, is this yearning for? At the time it felt like a desire to be close to the wolf, to be with him where he was. But what did that mean? I have not found an answer to this, but I have come to a place where it's alright to let the yearning be, even if I do not understand it. I have come to see it as an unexpected gift: as something that was sleeping in me that has wakened.

As I have learned to live with this yearning, I have noticed that it's tidal; it comes and goes in the pull of some deeper gravity. I see how it floods when I have been away from the land for too long, when I have been too much "in my head," too much in technology and information, too much in the city. I see how it ebbs at other times, such as when I look up into a night sky full of stars, or work in our yard, or when I stand outside at the start of the day with my eyes closed, and feel the morning's coolness on my face. I have come to understand that this yearning is not something I can satiate as I do my thirst. Rather, I notice that something paradoxical happens here. The more I drink this drink the greater my thirst; the greater my yearning. Could it be that the yearning is itself the connection I am yearning for?

THIRD

THE LAND

During the ten years I lived in my last home, from 2002 to 2012, I walked on the neighboring lands every day with our dogs in the morning and in the evening. I had read how a source of inspiration for Mary Oliver's poetry was her routine of walking the land near her home in Cape Cod, Massachusetts, day after day, year after year.[1] This encouraged me to approach the land and its inhabitants with attention and respect, and a willingness to be surprised.

Outside our gate was a perfectly manicured soccer field and to the south of this an area that had been left largely to itself. Its periphery was lined with live oaks; there was a central, open area of brush, to the east side of which was a cluster of non-native but nonetheless magnificent eucalyptus, where, one year, a pair of red-tailed hawks nested. At night, great horned owls and barn owls hunted there and in the morning we met coyotes on more than one occasion. A dirt road skirted all this, which is where we walked, the dogs and I, occasionally joined by Radhule, or by my young stepson, Ben, in what became an everyday practice. I began to keep a journal of some of my encounters on these daily walkabouts. Here are some extracts from the cycle of a year's turning on the land.

January

Out with dogs, on this misty morning. Milena with her smile and her one white, one blue Aussie eyes, and little Schnucks, with his shih tzu swagger and his floppy fringe. Such gladness coming onto this land. Seeing a black phoebe on a rock. Seeing mallards in the pond. And then a wave of house finches and their song. I pause, close my eyes, and open myself to the birdsong. I realize that in some ways John Moriarty's instruction to "Let nature happen to you"[2] is too big; too general. The instruction should be more specific. So, choose a particular aspect of the landscape that interests you, such as the song of the house finches, bring all your attention to that, and then, let the finches' song happen to you. Open your ears and your chest wide and let *finchsong happen to you.* Close your eyes, bring all your attention to the sensations of your face, and let the cool morning mist happen to you.

February

———

Walking on the land after the first rains in months. Everything washed, and fresh, and shining. Everything around me, everything on this land, comes into being through allowing. *Being through allowing.* Is-ness through allowing. Am-ness through allowing. Where sun meets leaf, being through allowing. Where rain meets earth, being through allowing. The unconditional surrender at the heart of it all. I stand before an oak and follow the flow of its trunk up into its highest branches. Words come: "I drink through my roots and am free."

March

———

A morning of birds. When walking with the dogs, I find a feather on the ground, small, mostly black, with a white band along the length of one side. I think it's black phoebe's feather. These days, on my runs, I meet him by his nest, where the overflow drain pool is below the soccer field. Later, as I arrive back at the house, I stop because right in front of my face is a little Allen's hummingbird. She must have been visiting the blossoms on the hedge at the side of the house. I pause, and at that moment, my body jumps, as this huge crow comes cawing in alarm with its wings flayed in a swoop, being chased by an angry mockingbird. Chase—flash—"CAW!"—swoop—flail—"CAASHHHH!" I stand there, wide awake now.

April

Out walking with the dogs this misty morning. Standing in front of the great eucalyptus trees in the mist, in their great silence, in their great abiding. Just being in their presence, seeing them, feeling their silence in my body, standing under them where all the little succulents are laid out and noticing the earth is wet and hearing the drops of moisture falling. This microclimate they are creating, these great-grandfathers, and these little ones. In their presence, something in me begins to flow. It's like walking among Buddhas. They are flow. Being in their presence, something in me begins to thaw, to soften, to liquefy, and, almost, to break into flame.

May

———

I look up at a flock of crows surfing on some currents of air and I think how birds are so aligned with the flow, as dolphins are with water.

Air is flow

Water is flow

Fire is flow.

And earth ... earth looks so solid but that's the grand illusion: our misconception is not to recognize that the Earth too is flow—just very, very, very slow flow.

June

———

As I step out of the gate in the morning, the sun is shining on the grass and on my heart, and the air is full of birds and birdsong.... It occurs to me that there is so much that we don't have to do. We don't have to make the sun shine. That's what the sun does. We don't have to make the birds sing. That's what they do. It's not all up to us. And yet, when we notice, when we pay attention, our participation makes a difference. Some mysterious alchemy happens when we bring our careful attention to what is.

July

Just now, out with the dogs, I pause by the corner in front of a brown swoop of grass still with some morning mist on it and low-rising sunlight catching it ever so lightly. As I stand there watching and waiting for Schnucks to catch up with us, I am able for a minute to appreciate the lightness of the light; how lightly the light touches the Earth. In this early morning, it's newborn. It makes me aware of a corresponding lightness in my heart that I have carried with me from my earlier meditation.

Later I am walking by the black phoebe's nest and watching out for snails on the ground. I see a clump of three of them together and another a little way apart, and I move to avoid them in my big boots. The dogs just walk straight through, either avoiding or touching them so lightly that the snails just carry on regardless. I realize that the dogs are walking lightly on the Earth without forethought, whereas I have to keep my eyes open and remain alert and attentive. Continually staying awake is a big part of what it takes for us humans to walk lightly on the Earth.

August

———

Coming out here this evening with the dogs, I notice that my heart is full of pain. I've just come home from a family meeting with a mother and her daughter. The mother had a massive stroke that left her paralyzed on her right side and unable to swallow. She's had a temporary feeding tube in for a couple of weeks now, but there has been no improvement and she's been told there's little chance of recovery. She just wants it all to end. She says she's had enough. She's ready. But her daughter is not. She's pregnant with her first child who is due in three-months' time. She wants her mother to accept a gastric feeding tube so she'll live long enough to see her grandchild. They're very close. They were both in tears as I sat with them.

I take off my shoes and begin to walk across the field. I look up and see a full moon rising through the eucalyptus. I stop to take a photo with my phone. As I do, a red-tailed hawk peels off the branches with a rolling screech and drops across the moon. I feel the coolness of the new cut grass with the soles of my feet.

September

———

As I am out with the dogs this evening, I notice an empty plastic water bottle on the ground. I go in under the branches of the oaks and pick it up. As I walk back across the field with it in my hand, I am thinking: *The land is so creative, and so powerful, and so capable in so many ways and yet here is one thing that she cannot do; she cannot pick up a plastic bottle off the ground.* But then I suddenly understand something. That yes she can! I am her capacity to do this. I am the land on two legs with the capacity to choose and to act.

October

When I come to the corner by the big oak this morning, there are two rabbits sitting in the sun. It seems to me that after night, after twelve hours of darkness, the homeostasis of the wild comes back again. The words of a haiku well up in my mind:

> After night,
> The wild is back again
> Like some great silent tide.

November

Coming out to the garden just now with the dogs, I notice movement on the ground to the left by the gate. It's a Bewick's wren feeding. In the past month, I have been seeing her more often. She has been here all these years but it's only now she's allowing me to see her. Watching her hopping and pecking her way toward me through the leaves with her banded tail perked up reminds me of the robin at Colman's Well. I show my respect by stepping out of her way.

I love this land that has, in some way, let me in. As I've walked here every day, I have got to know the black phoebe, and the juncos and the towhees, and the redtails, and the eucalyptus, and the great rock, and the crows, and the hummingbirds. It seems to me that the more familiar I've become with the beings that live here, the more I've been graced by their coming toward me. I know that I too belong here. I'm full of gratitude.

December

Waking up this morning, I realize that my "who-I-am-ness" is a co-arising of all the causes and conditions of this moment, including this land that I am living on and with. So, my "who-I-am-ness" is an open living system of presence that includes this place. In a sense, I am this place. And not just any place. I am this particular place with the sun coming through the mist before us as we walk through the gate, knowing that we will be leaving here soon, and stepping onto the dew-drenched grass. Breath and body, feeling and place, co-arising together.

* * *

The ritual of walking the land in this way every day was about becoming familiar with place. In his book *What the Robin Knows*, Jon Young shares the following San teaching from Africa:

> If one day I see a small bird and recognize it, a thin thread will form between me and that bird. If I just see it but don't really recognize it, there is no thin thread. If I go out tomorrow and see and really recognize that same individual small bird again, the thread will thicken and strengthen just a little. Every time I see and recognize that bird, the thread strengthens. Eventually it will grow into a string, then a cord, and finally a rope.... We make ropes with all aspects of the creation in this way.[3]

It was not just about noticing the birds; it was about noticing individual birds, for example, not just any black phoebe but that particular black phoebe who is always on his own, who nests by the drain pool; and individual trees, like the oak that stands by the corner with the children's swing on one of its branches; and particular rocks, like that great sandstone grandfather whose rust and ochre yellows deepen as the sun sets. We make relationships with these individuals one at a time.

Over time, I began to sense something else: that this place was becoming familiar with me. Wolf Wahpepah talks about how, when we walk out onto a landscape, we are "being regarded." How we carry ourselves, what our attitude is to a particular place and those who live there, is not going unobserved. If our attitude is one of respect, we may detect signs that this has been noticed. I began to recognize such signs, or at least I think I did, and not in dramatic ways but in little ways that could very easily have been overlooked. For example, the black phoebe allowed me to come closer to him before flying off, and then he would do so in a relaxed loop to a nearby branch rather than flying away fast in a straight line. Not infrequently, as I walked beneath the oaks, or the eucalyptus, or barefoot on the field, a quickening, an opening, happened within my experiencing that reminded me of Mary Oliver's description of coming into a sense of deep kinship with the land she walked daily:

> Eventually I began to appreciate—I don't say this lightly—that the great black oaks knew me. I don't mean they knew me as myself and not another—that kind of individualism was not in the air—but that they recognized and responded to my presence, and to my mood. They began to offer, or I began to feel them

offer, their serene greeting. It was like a quick change
of temperature, a warm and comfortable flush, faint
yet palpable....[4]

Jon Young talks about "invisibility" as one of the fruits of
deep nature connection.[5] By this he is not suggesting that we
learn to disappear. By invisibility he means that we become
so familiar to a particular landscape, we come to so deeply
belong there, that we no longer stand out as different and are,
therefore, no longer noticed. Toward the end of my time of living
on and with this land, I believe I experienced some moments of
invisibility.

The encounter I talked about earlier with the Bewick's
wren may have been one such occasion. Another was what
happened on my last morning in our previous home, when I
had wandered out into our backyard, early, to say my goodbyes.
There was a family of California quail there, which continued
to feed as I stood watching. They were relaxed and feeding from
the ground while gently companion-calling back and forth to
one another. After a little while, a young female started moving
in my direction, pecking as she came. She continued coming,
closer and closer towards where I was standing, now just a foot
or two away, as if she did not see me. Just as I was thinking,
"Maybe I've become so at home in this yard that I'm not visible
to her; maybe she is going to come right up to me..." she lifted

her head and saw me. All at once she startled, gave an alarm call and flew off in a panic, almost crashing into the cabin at the side of the yard. I thought about this afterward and asked myself if indeed I had been "invisible," or if this was just one very preoccupied adolescent grouse?

FOURTH

THE NEST IN THE STREAM

Wolf and Lisa smudged us down with the smoke from a smoldering stem of dried white sage and gave each of us a glass of water and a pinch of tobacco to take with us. They instructed us to go silently out onto the land and to walk about looking for a place where we would like to spend some time. I made my way down to a creek among the trees to the east. I found a spot that was secluded and accessible, and with some awkwardness, because of having no free hands to steady myself, descended the steep, dry, leaf-covered creek side to the water's edge.

At first I just stood there, looking at the rocks in the creek bed upstream and watching and listening as the water flowed around them. I was standing at a place where the stream broadens into a pool. Looking down, I noticed that the water at my feet was utterly still and clear, reflecting the blues and greens of what was overhead, but there was something else.

There was something unusual, partially submerged in the water. Small branches, twigs in a swirl. It was a large bird's nest. I instinctively looked up into the branches of the sycamore tree above me.

When I found a spot where I could safely leave the tobacco and water, I walked to where there were some stepping stone-like rocks going across the creek. I was able to squat down on one of these and look back into the pool. I was directly downstream of the nest. As I looked more closely, I could see that it was perfectly intact. It could not have been in the water very long because there were still pieces of wool interwoven with the twigs. The weave of the nest appeared loose yet solid. There were spaces between some of the coils and I could tell the water was flowing through as fine threads of what looked like hair or grass were waving lazily at its lower edge.

As I squatted there, looking at the nest with the water flowing through, I became aware of a loosening in my torso and limbs. I imagined water flowing through me. I felt like I was being washed clean, as though I were letting go of something heavy that I had been carrying around for a long time.

Before I left, I poured the glass of water on the ground and dropped the tobacco in the stream in gratitude. When I returned, Wolf and Lisa and everyone else were already sitting in a circle under the oaks. We each shared our stories. The image of the nest in the stream, with the water flowing through it, and the phrase "the loose and open weave of the heart" stayed with me all through that night.

The nest in the stream speaks to me of a way of being that is deeply receptive. Our hearts pump, but only after they have opened their atria wide to receive the body's blood. Receptivity is neither a feminine nor a masculine quality. It is how our heart is in its most relaxed state. Our hearts are designed to receive before they pump, and our lives depend on this happening.

It is important to distinguish between receptivity and passivity. Passivity suggests defeat and may have negative connotations, especially to those who have been on the receiving end of abusive power relationships. Receptivity, on the other hand, implies a conscious choice. Choosing an attitude of receptivity, choosing to open our hearts wide, and to keep them open, even in the face of suffering, is a courageous and powerful way of meeting the world.

John Moriarty speaks eloquently about this. He describes this stance as "A new kind of heroism." He says, "A hero like Cuchulainn isn't what we need. We need another kind of hero altogether.... A hero now isn't someone who goes out and fights the sea.... The hero now isn't someone who wields a sword—it's someone who puts down his sword and lets nature happen to him."[1] The new kind of hero is one who faces life with an open and receptive heart.

In watching the nest in the stream, I began to understand

the relationship between receptivity and compassionate action. As the heart opens, receives, and swells, before it pumps, so the impulse to act is born in receptivity. When we come into the state of being that is deep receptivity, the impulse for compassionate action emerges, spontaneously. Bernie Glassman, author and founder of Zen Peacemakers, writes:

> When we bear witness, when we become the situation—homelessness, poverty, illness, violence, death—the right action arises by itself. We don't have to worry about what to do. We don't have to figure out solutions ahead of time. Peacemaking is the function of bearing witness. Once we listen with our entire body and mind, loving action arises.[2]

I am reminded of a teaching from my root tradition that continues to be full of significance for me. The angel Gabriel has just announced to the Virgin Mary that she is to give birth to a child who will be the messiah for whom Israel is waiting. I imagine Mary pausing. I imagine her head saying, "That's impossible!" and her heart saying, "What if?" I imagine her confusion. I imagine the moment that she chooses to trust as she opens to the silence between the words, and I hear her reply, "Let what you have said be done unto me." In consciously opening to the flow of what is, the miraculous happens.

The nest in the stream brings me into a new sense of self. I had always considered myself to have substance and solidity, and despite the changes that came with time, a certain continuity and permanence. Now, as I watched the stream flowing through the nest, I began to understand that this is not how it is. On their own, the nest is just a nest and the stream is just a stream. Together, they form an image of temporary solidity in fluidity. I realize that I too am a transient pattern in change, and I wonder if this is what the Buddha meant when he spoke of "no-self" and "impermanence": that while there is "no-*separate-solid-permanent*-self" there is self-as-change, self-as-relationship; self-as-flow-through.

Above all, the nest in the stream teaches me a new way of being with pain; my own, the pain of others, and our world's. I have come to see that there are different elements to this teaching that interweave with one another. The first of these is that the nest is *in* the stream. The nest is not in the branches of the sycamore above the stream, where, in a sense, it belongs. It's in the stream, which is unusual and like an out-of-context dream image, calls particular attention to itself. The nest in the stream shows me how I am inextricably connected with the rest of nature. It speaks of how, in my deepest identity, I am immersed in the flow of life. The nest's being in the stream tells me that it begins by my realizing this, by my remembering this, by my experiencing this.

When I look more closely, I see that the water is flowing *through* the nest. I recognize this is only possible because the nest itself, how it is structured, allows this to happen. The teaching I receive here is about opening to the pain that I am feeling; not just being present to it, but consciously, and as deliberately as a buffalo with an approaching storm, turning to face it, head on, and, as I do this, letting it flow into me. As the water continues to flow through the nest, I understand this is not just about being receptive to the pain but also about allowing myself to feel it. This is about experiencing in my body what Eugene Gendlin calls "the felt sense" of the pain.[3] This is about suffering my suffering.

When I step back, I notice the bigger, deeper stream that is flowing over and between the rocks upstream and downstream and to either side of the nest. I see that the essence of the stream is in its always flowing; it's always flowing through. And, as I see this, I hear an invitation not to cling to my pain, not to ruminate on the narrative of who is to blame and what this pain is about, but instead, to return, again and again if necessary, to the felt-sense of the pain, and then, *to release it*, to surrender it, to let it go, to the always flowing through of the deeper stream.

Finally, as I expand my awareness further still, I see that the stream is flowing into the river, and the river is flowing into the ocean, and the ocean is rising as clouds, and the clouds are falling as rain, and that the rain has, once again, become the stream; that all is flow, that all is flowing-through. I understand then what Wolf means when he says that pain is energy, and the energy that is our pain does not belong to us; when we unconditionally release our pain to the Earth, we are releasing energy back into the great creative cycling that is life. I see now that I do not have to hold onto my pain, that I can let it go to the deeper stream, and I can do so in the hope it may be of benefit to others in a way I cannot see or imagine, and will never know.

What this looks like in practice is that I begin by paying attention to the breath, to the sensations of the breath stream, which allows me to experience the flow of inner nature connection. It means honoring whatever pain I am feeling just then, by letting it be as it is, not trying to change it in any way. It means opening to the pain with the inhale, and for just a few moments, lingering with the felt-sense of the pain in my body, however I am registering it. Then—and this is especially challenging for me—it means unconditionally releasing the pain, letting it go with the exhale, to the bigger, deeper flowing through.

The other day I sat with a young woman, Jo, who is dying of ovarian cancer. She was feeling very fatigued and was frustrated by this and her lack of independence. As I was sitting by her bedside in her room the hospice, I looked out the window at the coastal oaks, at the hummingbirds coming to drink at the nearby fountain, the juncos picking on the ground nearby, and among the branches of the oak, the blueness of the sky. I mused out loud how wonderful it would be if we could just plug into this incredibly creative, interflowing, co-arising energy that is nature. I told Jo how I found that sometimes the simple act of paying attention to other-than-human nature with all my senses enabled me to do this. When I had finished speaking, she looked at me in silence for a few seconds. Then she said, "No offense, but I think that's bullshit."

I smarted at this, and pulled back into myself. I struggled to find my feet, and my voice. I acknowledged to Jo that I understood that my approach may not be her way. I asked her what energized her, what restored her spirit. How and where did she find peace in times of chaos? Jo began to talk about her daughter, with whom she was very close. "If only she would spend more time with me. It seems to be too hard for her. I guess she's doing the best she can," she said.

As I listened, I felt for Jo in her loneliness and grief. I was aware that I still had some hurt feelings from being rebuffed in my earlier attempts to help. I brought my awareness inwards to the sensations of my breath. Then I turned my awareness to what I was feeling, and for a few moments, I allowed myself to experience what this felt like in my body. Breathing in, I opened up; breathing out, I consciously let my feelings of discomfort go. I continued to breathe in this way; opening with the inhale, letting go with the exhale. Jo was quietly weeping now. I reached out with my left hand and placed it on her foot. For a little while, we sat there like that in silence.

Once again, I see how frightened I am of pain and how I have always done everything I can to avoid it. My career of "managing pain" has allowed me to come close to the suffering of others but always from a position of power and expertise. I see how, over time, I have paid a price for this. The short-term comfort of being protected from what was messy and uncomfortable has given way over time to a pervasive sense of disconnection and isolation and, with this, low-grade unhappiness and burnout.

The nest in the stream offers a radically different teaching. It suggests that I do not have to be so defended any more. It offers me a way of holding my pain that is not so self-protective. "Let suffering happen to you," it whispers. "Allow it in. Feel it as it washes through. And then, let it go to the deeper flow of life. This will bring you out of isolation and into connection."

When we are in pain, we tend to pull back, to contract, to cut off, to curl up in a ball and separate ourselves from others. But pain in isolation is the definition of suffering. Pain that is trapped in an isolated system, such as when we are ruminating on our hurt feelings, is perpetuating itself, and only making things worse. The paradoxical teaching of the nest in the stream is that turning toward, opening to, feeling with, and then letting go of our pain brings us back into connection, back into relationship, back into an open living system—and this changes everything.

I can see how the nest in the stream could, at first glance, appear to be the wrong medicine for someone who already feels overwhelmed by pain. After all, the prescription involves opening to, allowing in, and being with what already feels like "too much." But pain that we resist, or that we try to contain with our own effort, intensifies and becomes an even greater threat.

The key is in our capacity to choose. Jung says, "Don't drown. Dive!"[4] By choosing to open to and experience my pain, and by then choosing to release my pain to the flowing through, I paradoxically find myself empowered rather than weakened. Yes, at first I may feel the pain more intensely than I did before, but then I notice a subtle yet significant change; the pain has somehow lost its sting, and I am now more awake, more alive, and more connected.

As I learn from the nest in the stream that my deeper identity is to be a flow-through to life, with all that this brings, I experience a lightness of being. Before, it felt as though it was all up to me. It was my responsibility to manage someone else's pain in whatever way I could, and that brought a certain heaviness on on my shoulders. The nest in the stream teaches me that while it is still my responsibility to do what I can to help and to hold another's pain, my even greater charge is to be with my own pain, and, ultimately, to surrender the energy that is my pain to the deeper currents that are flowing through my life, in the hope that this will somehow be of benefit to others. It is such a relief to know that it's not all up to me. I still do all I can to ease others' pain. I still suffer my suffering in the face of another's pain, but it does not end there. I do what I do in the spirit and practice of letting be and letting go to the flowing through that I am immersed in and that is happening naturally, without any volition on my part, and without an expectation of a particular outcome.

This morning as I was out running, I noticed as if for the first time how much harder it is to run uphill than it is to run downhill. I thought, "This is because, when I'm running downhill, I'm running with gravity. That's what makes it easier." With this thought I flashed back to the nest in the stream, and saw that the water would not be flowing through without gravity; gravity is the invisible dynamic of the nest in the stream.

Surrendering to gravity allows life to flow through us. At the deepest level, we don't have to do anything. The water is already flowing through *all by itself*. The flowing through is how it is, how we are, in our deepest nature. What we can do is to wake up to this, to remember this, and with our great yes, to consciously realign ourselves with what is already happening. As we do this, we open the floodgates of compassion as we too become nests in the stream.

In the weeks after this encounter, I went back occasionally to visit the creek and to check to see if the nest was still there.

Each time I did, I found it more waterlogged and worn. It had by then sunk to the bottom of the pool and the coils of twigs were bare. Eventually, the few remaining bigger weaves began to loosen and fall apart, until one day when I visited, the pool was empty.

FIFTH

UP ON THE HILL

Wolf and Lisa describe the vision quest as the most "intensely personal" of all Native American ceremonies. How the vision quest is conducted varies with different traditions. What is common to all is that the ceremony involves a time of waiting and fasting on the land, alone, while "crying for a vision."

After attending sweat lodge ceremonies for some time, I offered Wolf tobacco and asked him if he would consider putting me "up on the hill" on vision quest. We spoke for a while about why I wanted to do this. I said, "I have a longing in my heart to be close to the Earth." He looked at me silently for a few moments before we shook hands as he accepted the pouch of tobacco I was offering.

With Wolf and Lisa's detailed instructions, I prepared for my vision quest with a group of five others over the following six months. The preparation included making a specified number of "prayer-ties"—pinches of tobacco in small squares of cotton—in each of the colors of the four directions. Each tie was made while burning sage and offering an individual prayer intention. Later, the prayer-ties would be laid out sun-wise on a bed of mountain sage to surround me during my time on the hill.

I was nervous about the fasting: no food or water for four days. Previous experience with kidney stones and my medical training told me that this may not be the smartest thing to do. I was reassured when Lisa later told me that she and Wolf, and their elders, had supported a great many vision quests for two generations without any mishap. She pointed out that ordinary people have been doing this for thousands of years. Wolf added, "If it's too hard, you come down. But the fasting is important. It's what drives the prayer."

The day before going on the hill, I gathered mountain sage in the high desert with my fellow questers, to be used as groundcover in our "altar," the small rectangular space marked by four willow staffs at each corner where we would be during our fast. This was a day of eating and drinking and making last-minute preparations. It included instruction from Wolf and Lisa on how to tie the six, large prayer-ties called "prayer flags," and a special prayer flag called "The Red Blanket." As we worked, Wolf told us, "The flags are powerful offerings to the grandfathers of the four directions, and to Mother Earth, and Father Sky. An especially powerful spirit is attracted to the Red

Blanket. That particular spirit only has permission to pick up prayers that affect large groups of individuals. It's a prayer for the people."

At sunrise the following morning, Wolf led us in two rounds of a "dust off" sweat. This was a deliberately mild sweat so we would not lose body water as we began our fast. We six vision questers were in the honor seat in the west, directly opposite the door. Wolf was sitting at his usual spot just north of the door. He told us: "During life there's a cord of connection between body and spirit, but at the moment of death the cord is severed. If it's a sudden death the cord breaks abruptly. If it's a gradual death it's a more lingering process; then the cord gradually disintegrates with little pieces breaking off over time. This attracts the attention of the ancestors."

"When you begin your fast," Wolf continued, "You're beginning the dying process. As far as I know, we two-leggeds are the only animals that voluntarily choose to give up water. So we enter this dying state in order to attract the attention of the spirits. We have been doing it this way for thousands of years because it works and because we don't know of a better way of coming into that state of being we call prayer. The spirits pay attention. They come and notice what's going on. There's a spirit to attend to each of your prayer-ties."

Before we had entered the lodge, we had filled our sacred pipes and left them on the altar outside. As we left the lodge, we were instructed to pick up our sacred pipe and to hold its red bowl in our left hand to our chest, while holding the stem in our right hand pointing diagonally upward and away. We were then led the mile or so into the backcountry to our altars. Wolf came to where I was kneeling on the ground in my altar with the sacred pipe in my hands. He put a blanket around me and then, squatting beside me with an arm around my shoulder, he said a prayer for me and left.

I was on my own. Slowly I looked around. I was in a grove of scrub oaks through which I could glimpse the mountains on the far side of the valley. Holding my sacred pipe, I knelt on a bed of mountain sage surrounded on all sides by the hundreds of brightly colored prayer-ties. It was exquisitely beautiful. After all the months of preparation, I had arrived. A wave of exhaustion swept through me. I laid the sacred pipe on the altar, a small mound of sage in the corner, unrolled my sleeping bag, and crawled into it. I slept for several hours.

That was Wednesday morning and I was already twelve hours into my four-day fast. My Red Blanket prayer was that I would come to see more clearly what I could best do to serve our Mother Earth for the sake of the future generations.

I prayed a lot. I always began by honoring the six directions. One at a time and moving clockwise, I engaged with the landscape in each direction through my five senses. Closing my eyes, I noticed whatever sounds were coming toward me.

Opening my eyes, I took in the light, the textures, the colors, the movements. Closing my eyes, I paid attention to the touch of the breeze or the temperature on my skin. Opening my mouth, I tasted the air, which was especially beautiful in the cool of early morning or late at night. Eyes still closed and lifting my chin, I sniffed the air several times briskly, and inhaled the smells of the dried brush and the mountain sage. Next, I opened my eyes again, and holding my sacred pipe, bent my knees and touched the earth with my other hand. I stood, and looking upward, stretched my hand toward the sky. Then, pressing the bowl of the sacred pipe against my heart, I bent my head, closed my eyes, and remembered why I was there.

I spent a lot of time sitting on my rolled-up sleeping bag, looking around and noticing what was happening. I knew that the most respectful way I could be present in this place was to be open and receptive by paying attention and really listening. The animals came. Chipmunk. Rabbit. And the birds. There was a small brown bird who had the sweetest song I ever heard. She hung around in the scrub oaks for what seemed like a long time. A western tanager came. His startling yellows and reds somehow quenched my thirst for a little while. There were mountain grouse in the eastern meadow and this one particular little guy with a tassel on his head who jumped up in the air again and again, plucking at grass seeds. He would appear suddenly from behind the grasses as he leapt into the air, then disappear as he came back to earth, only to immediately reappear as if bouncing on a hidden trampoline. Watching and being watched. Noticing and being noticed. There was something beautifully matter-of-fact about it all. It was not a big deal. It was just how it was to be with my relations in the natural world.

It was Friday morning, forty-eight hours into the fast. I was sitting on my rolled-up sleeping bag holding my sacred pipe. I noticed some movement on the sleeping pad. I looked more closely and saw a cluster of ants milling around and attacking a ladybug that was on its back. I hesitated, not knowing if it was the right thing to intervene but decided to do so. As gently as I could I picked up the tiny, lifeless red and black spotted body between my thumb and index fingers and put it on a small stone on my sage altar. I left her there in the warm sun to see if she would recuperate a little bit and regain her strength. I sat with my sacred pipe watching her. After lying completely still for some time, she began to move. It was though she had been under the anesthetic of the ant venom but was now recovering. Then she began moving her legs and flicked open her wings as if she was about to take off. A sudden movement in my peripheral vision caught my attention. Another ladybug had flown in and landed on the altar. Then another one came, then another, then another. Some flew into the cooled ash from the burnt sage in the abalone shell on the altar, and crawled around in there. A few of them came and landed right on me. The first one landed on the back of my left hand. As I slowly lifted my hand toward my face, she flew off. But then another ladybug landed on my right forearm; then another on my right thigh. At one time, I counted ten ladybugs on the backs of my hands, my arms, my legs, and the front of my chest and belly. I looked back at the one I had rescued. She was still flexing her opened wings. Then she flew off and, one by one, the others followed.

Later that afternoon I felt a deep longing. I began to weep. I prayed, "Is there something I need to see, is there something I need to hear?" As I cried, I was holding the bowl of the sacred pipe to my heart, while resting my forehead on the stem, which I held in the way I had been taught. Then, as naturally as the birdsong in the nearby scrub oak, I was aware of words arising in the silence of my heart: *"You are one of us now ..."*

I was surprised and yet not surprised. It was as though my body recognized this voice. I felt a loosening in my chest and sensed an effortless falling back into place.

The next morning was time to end my fast and I was ready and waiting from first light, holding my sacred pipe. I heard drumming and Lisa's approaching singing. I began to weep. Lisa came to my altar and said, "Relative, it's time to come home now." She led me and the other five vision questers back to camp.

Sitting by the fire, one at a time we vision questers smoked our sacred pipes in silence. After a few puffs we each passed our sacred pipe to Wolf and Lisa who, in turn, passed it on clockwise to the circle of relatives and supporters, inviting them to share. We were then offered our first drink of water in four days. It hurt my throat as it went down. We next shared three bowls of sacred foods: sweet corn, minced meat, and berries. As we ate, Wolf told us that the meat we were eating was buffalo meat, with pine nuts, no seasoning, but slow cooked and really soft so that the elders, without teeth, could eat it. He said, "We learned this from the animals. We watched how the wolf chewed food for her pups and toothless elders and spat it out for them. We learned this from the wolf." Then he added, "Animals civilize us...."

After this we crawled into the lodge for two rounds of a dust-off sweat. These two rounds were the closing to the opening rounds we had had at the start of the vision quest four days earlier. When we crawled out, Wolf turned to our families and friends around the fire and said, "They're back. Now you can greet your loved ones."

"You are one of us now." I have asked myself many times since then what these words could mean. Whose words were they? Even now, several years later, I still don't know. It does not seem to matter. What does matter is that in some way I felt I was being welcomed into a bigger family, and that this was the beginning of an answer to the question I had been holding in my Red Blanket prayer. I was, and continue to be, deeply honored to have been blessed in this way.

Two teachings of Wolf's helped me to appreciate the significance of what had happened here. The first was when he talked about the nature of "visions." He said, "A vision is anything that helps you to realize something more about yourself or the nature of reality. Of course, it might be an external vision but it could also be an insight, or a voice, or a visit, or a synchronicity, or a medicine dream… What matters is not so much the form it takes as that it deepens your understanding of reality." The second was on an occasion when he was talking about hummingbirds. He had spoken about how hummingbirds were one of the smallest and sweetest expressions of the power of the Thunder Beings that live in the sky and bring thunder and lightning and rain. He had added, "When they come in this form [as these smallest of birds], we're not afraid; they allow us to come close to them."

The robin at Colman's Well, the wolf on the road in Yellowstone, the many meetings on the land by our home, the nest in the stream, even if unusual, were, objectively, ordinary events that I had subjectively experienced as extraordinary. In contrast, what had happened with the ladybugs was, objectively, an event out of the ordinary. For them to come to me as they had was beyond the realm of "mere coincidence." Even if this was a very small-scale event, it was a powerful synchronicity. Wolf says, "Indian way, we see two unconnected events coinciding in a meaningful manner as the work of the spirits. They are breadcrumbs the Creator is leaving for us to follow." He added, "We Indians don't believe in miracles; we rely on them."

We cannot make synchronicities happen. What we can do, as the vision quest ceremony taught me, is to create the conditions that make it more likely that they will occur. Synchronicities arise from a participatory process between us and the natural environment. Here this meant lying on the Earth long enough, in solitude and silence, fasting and praying, while watching, and waiting, and listening, for my pulse to come into some deeper harmony. An attitude of respect, coupled with deep connection with the living landscape, make it more likely that such events will occur, and that we will recognize them when they do.

There is a curious addendum to this story. Yesterday, as I lunched with a friend, I told her this story. Afterward, I returned to the meadow where I was writing. My plan was to spend the afternoon working on this story. As I approached my blue canvas seat I noticed a bright red dot; there was a ladybug on it.

SIXTH

THE TREE OF LIFE

In the spring of 2013 I talked to Wolf and Lisa about the possibility of going to that summer's Sun Dance ceremony as a supporter, and they invited me to join them. I had been hearing about the Sun Dance for some time and felt a growing desire to go. It seemed like the right time.

The Sun Dance ceremony is one of the most sacred ceremonies of the Plains Indians and is now practiced by many Native American tribes. Some Sun Dance ceremonies also welcome non-Natives to pray in this way. At the heart of the ceremony is the sacrifice the dancers make. They fast from food and water for four days and four nights, as they dance in an enclosure called "the arbor" around a specially chosen cottonwood tree. They willingly take on suffering in this way for their loved ones but also, as Wolf says, "for the benefit of all life that relies on the Earth, and the Earth herself."

On that first night at the Sun Dance grounds, I and some other first-timers met with an elder who talked to us about the ceremony. He said, "It's hard to know what to say to you newcomers about the dance... What I can say is that it's the most beautiful thing I have ever done in my life." A little later he added, "Some people say we come here to suffer. We don't come here to suffer. We come here to pray, and to heal."

The following day, as we sat together in our community kitchen after breakfast, Wolf spoke to us about what would happen later that day, called "Tree Day," the day preceding the four days of the dance.

"We call Sun Dance 'suffering for the people,'" he began. "The warriors decided that this was a way they could help the people. Sun Dance is a give-away ceremony from the warriors to the people. During this time of offering, the dancers want to take upon themselves everything that hurts the people. Anything that causes the people misery is considered to be 'the enemy.' So the Chief will say to his helpers, 'Go find the enemy and when you find him come back and tell me where he is.' Then the helpers go out and look for a tree. It has to be a cottonwood tree and it must have certain characteristics. That tree represents the enemy, all that's hurting the people, and that's why we need to capture it and bring it back to camp."

Later that morning everyone in camp made the journey to a nearby forest where the scouts had found "the enemy." The cottonwood tree whose life was about to be taken was tall and slender; its thickest branches reached up like two great arms through the canopy into the sun. The little girls who made the first blows with the axe were so young and sweet. It began with their gentleness and innocence. After them it was the elders' turn. I looked up at the highest branches and noticed a red-tailed hawk circling clockwise, right overhead, around and around. I saw that others noticed this too but no one seemed surprised. As we carried the tree down through the camp and into the arbor and laid it sideways on some wooden trestles to prevent it from touching the ground, the big drum singers started. Then, all the people came into the arbor with prayer-ties they had prepared beforehand and tied them to the branches of the tree, so that they would directly benefit from the sacrifice of the dancers.

Back in camp that night, Wolf spoke to us again.

"Now, the dance will begin tomorrow. The people are very grateful to the dancers because they're the ones making the sacrifice. All we have to do is bring our prayers. We're told that as soon as that tree goes up, and all the details have been arranged as we were instructed, it transforms. It's no longer 'the enemy,' as soon as it goes up, it becomes 'the Tree of Life.'

"We're told that the Creator, the Great Mystery, comes and enters that tree and will stand there, right in front of us, for four days so that we can walk right up to him and tell him what we need. Someone once said to me, 'Don't you people understand that the Creator, God, is everywhere?' I said, 'Yes, of course the answer is yes, but when something is everywhere, it's really hard to approach.' So the Creator gave us a ceremony where we could just walk right up to him."

Early the following morning I stood at the edge of the arbor with the hundred or so other supporters who were there. As I looked around the circular clearing at the center of the forest, I saw how everyone was standing in silent anticipation. In front of us were small, painted willow sticks with red tobacco prayer-ties at their tips marking out the inner circle of the arbor, where only the Sun Dancers, the Chief and his helpers could enter. At the very center of the arbor was the Tree of Life, standing tall, its branches filled with hundreds of bright prayer-ties, its leaves still fresh and olive green. At four points around the circle of red willow sticks were large willow poles with big prayer flags in each of the colors of the different directions. Behind us, at the back of the arbor, an awning roofed with leafed branches would offer some shade later in the day for the supporters. In the background, surrounding the Tree of Life, rose a circle of great trees, some hundreds of feet high—cottonwoods, cedars, big-leaf maples, bitter cherries, Douglas firs, red alder, and western hemlock.

An opening to the east, the East Gate, was flanked on both sides by two young girls, each holding the handles of canisters filled with burning sacred herbs. Smoke billowed upward in the morning air. Just as the sun rose above the tree line, the big drum singers started to play. With this, a procession began to enter through the East Gate. At the front came the head male helper carrying the buffalo skull, followed by the head female helper carrying the main sacred pipe of the Sun

Dance ceremony. She was flanked on either side by helpers carrying eagle staffs, who were followed by more helpers. Then came twenty or so male and female dancers and, at the end of the procession, the Chief. The Sun Dance had begun.

It was the evening of the first day of the dance. As I sat outside my tent to write in my journal, I found that I had no words to describe adequately what I had witnessed that day. It was by then beginning to get dark and I could still hear the big drum and the singing voices and the eagle whistles in the wind and trees overhead. I recalled how, during the breaks between the rounds of the day's dancing, the dancers had passed out their sacred pipes to the supporters at the edge of the arbor, who then sat to share the pipes in small circles on the ground. The dancers had sacrificed for the people; their dancing had made the prayers in their sacred pipes strong, and now these prayers were making the people strong.

As I lay down to sleep, I thought back on the day. That elder was right, what lingered was how beautiful it all was—the dancing, the drumming, the singing, the colors, the courage, the generosity, the gentleness, the fierceness; and all around, the great swaying trees that encircled the arbor. The first of the piercings came vividly to mind. I saw one of the Chief's helpers leading a male dancer to a buffalo robe on the ground. All around the arbor the dancing continued and the air was full of drumming and singing. The dancer lay there immobile on his back as the Chief threaded two sharp bone pins through the skin on either side of his chest. When the dancer stood up, the Chief placed the looped ends of two ropes around each pin. The other ends of the ropes were tied to the Tree of Life. The dancer moved backwards until the ropes tightened and the skin was pulled taut. By now he too was dancing, arms pumping and lifting alternate knees high in the air to the beat of the big drum as the ropes tugged on the bone pins, stretching his skin to a peak, as he, and all the other dancers, some already pierced, some not, blew loudly on their eagle whistles.

I spent the second day with other supporters at the edge of the arbor. While some sat resting in the shade, others began to dance. I joined in, lifting my arms and feet in rhythm with the pulse of the big drum. As the day went by, I noticed that my feet had worn two grooves into the ground. With each step, dust came up between my toes. It felt so good to have my feet in the earth in this way. As I danced, I watched the Tree of Life. Its leaves were already looking crinkled and paler than they had been and contrasted sharply with the deep, vibrant green of the trees behind and all around. It was as though, with the pulse of every drumbeat, the Tree of Life was becoming more transparent, more translucent, more porous. It had begun its fast at the same time as the dancers had theirs. The dancers and the tree were in this together.

In the breaks between the rounds, I lay on the ground and rested. During each of these breaks, an elder was invited to come into the arbor to share his or her story. I was deeply touched by how this community held its elders in such respect. When one of them spoke, everyone listened to what they had to say. One elder talked about humility as the basis of real power. "Think of the Earth," he said, "Its medicine comes from receiving all that dies into it. And the ocean," he continued, "its strength comes from receiving the rain and the rivers that flow into it." His face was beaming as he came out of the arbor to rejoin the supporters, carrying one of the dancer's sacred pipes. As I sat in a circle with him and some others to smoke the pipe, I marveled at how elders thrive when they are given their place in the sacred hoop and valued as the wisdom keepers that they are.

On the third day of the Sun Dance, I was standing with other supporters in the arbor, praying and dancing with the dancers. As I watched the ropes between the Tree of Life and the pierced eagle dancers, I realized that there were also invisible ropes going from the Tree of Life to everyone in the circle around the arbor, and in turn, other invisible ropes that went from each of us to those beyond us, and beyond, and beyond. I understood that just as these invisible ropes were connecting us to the Tree of Life, so too they were connecting the Tree of Life to us, and that energy was flowing in both directions, from each of us to the tree as prayer, and from the tree to each of us as blessing. Again I noticed, that as the vitality of the Tree of Life was ebbing day by day, hour by hour, as its leaves were becoming more anemic and shriveled, the great green brothers and sisters of the Tree Nation behind and all around were growing livelier and, it seemed to me, moving closer. In some mysterious way, the surrounding trees had also entered the great and sacred exchange that is the Sun Dance. I asked myself, "Is this what the heart of the world looks like?" That night my sleep was filled with song and eagle whistles and the beat of the big drum.

On the fourth day of the dance, I went down to the arbor early and sat there waiting. I watched as a robin landed on the grass, hunting for worms. He found one and flew off with the worm in his mouth. He landed briefly on the yellow prayer flag where he swallowed the worm before flying into the trees. Then, just as the sun came over the tops of the trees and into the arbor, the headman and headwoman, followed by the Chief and the other helpers, led the dancers in through the East Gate one last time, carrying the buffalo skull and the Sun Dance pipe to lay on the altar in the west. As the dancing began, I was filled with gratitude to have been part of this beautiful prayer and for all I had received. I looked up and saw the Tree of Life, standing at the center of the sacred hoop, holding the prayers of all the people and, in some mysterious way, united with everything in creation. The words "sacred connection" came to me. I saw that connection is not something we do or make but who we already are in our deepest nature. I understood then that this is what Wolf calls "our original instructions," meaning who and how the Creator intends us to be, and that as and when we remember this, we return to the state of being that is prayer.

The Sun Dance is a ceremony of deep remembering. The Sun Dance helps us to remember that we too are relatives, and why this matters. As Wolf puts it, "when we remember who we are, we know what's important, and when we know what's important, then we know what we have to do." Just as the ceremony helps us to remember who we are, perhaps, in some way, it also helps the rest of nature to remember who we are.

All through those four days of Sun Dance, the Tree of Life was at the center of the sacred hoop. As I looked at it now on this final day of the dance, I sensed that besides the cords of connection, some visible, some not, coming out from the Tree of Life to us two-legged humans, there were also roots of connection going out from the Tree of Life to the great Tree Nation surrounding us on all sides. The thought occurred to me that perhaps the Tree of Life had mediated a truce between our two nations. For hundreds of years, we humans had looked at trees only through economic eyes, as lumber to be cut down and sold, and not as the living, sentient beings they are. I could understand how the Tree Nation, seeing how preoccupied we were with doing our own thing and going our own way, could have have decided to carry on without us. But now I imagined the Tree Nation hearing the singing and the drumming and the eagle whistles, looking over their shoulders and seeing that we humans were dancing in a spirit of humility, and grief, and gratitude, and noticing that we were suffering for the people, and that when we approached the Tree of Life we did so with tenderness and reverence. And I pictured that great forest, realizing that we humans had remembered our ancient friendship, slowly, slowly turning, and once again joining in the dance.

More than once as I watched the eagle dancers "suffering for the people," I thought of the Buddhist hero figure of the *bodhisattva*, the one who, even though she or he has reached full enlightenment and could enter the eternal bliss of *nirvana*, chooses instead to turn around and reenter *samsara*, the world of suffering, and does this again, and again, and again, until all beings are happy, until all beings are safe, until all beings are free. The *bodhisattva* knows that the way to bring happiness, safety, and freedom to the people is to suffer with them: that this delivers them from the pain of separateness and brings them into the healing of community.

As I danced with them, I knew what Holocaust survivor Viktor Frankl meant when he quoted German philosopher Friedrich Nietzsche: "He who has a why to live can bear almost any how."[1] A sense of meaning makes it possible to bear the unbearable. The dancers could take the four days of fasting, the skin piercings, and the dancing in the sun beyond exhaustion, knowing that they were doing this for their people, for all people. The dancers' yearning to help the people was stronger than their pain. Once again, I understood that the deeper our connections are with others, the more we care about them. The more we care about them, the more we want to act, to do all that we can to help them, no matter what the cost.

Beauty and community are powerful containers of suffering. When I saw an exhausted Sun Dancer slump to his knees at the end of the dance and lean forwards to touch his forehead to the Earth, I flashed back to that time in my life when I was grieving the loss of contact with my daughters and I had collapsed on the floor, on the wolf robe, and found some comfort there. I remembered John, whom I had met many years before at St Christopher's Hospice, who had said to me, in words of surprise and relief, "The pain is still there, but I can live with it now." In the silent equanimity of nature, everyone and everything has a place.

After the closing ceremonies, as I was walking back to camp, a soft rain began to fall. I remembered something I had heard Wolf say about one of the Sun Dance songs we had just been singing. He had told us that the words of the song translated as "I will always be standing here to defend and protect Mother Earth." He had added, "In truth we're only here for four days and yet we'll always be standing here. Wherever we go, we'll still be standing here. We'll remember and we'll live this way."

After returning home, my weekly attendance at Wolf and Lisa's Monday night sweat lodge ceremonies helped me to stay in touch with what I had experienced at the Sun Dance. Even though this often left me a little sleep-deprived, I walked through Tuesdays with my feet sinking a little deeper into the earth and my heart a little more open to my patients' pain. As I walked my dogs in the mornings and noticed how the California towhee pair did not seem so alarmed at my approach and continued with their feeding—scratching, jumping back, pecking at whatever bug they had uncovered, and taking their time before moving on—I knew that there were cords here too, maybe fine and slender ones, but every bit as vital as those between the eagle dancers and the Tree of Life.

SEVENTH

POLARIS

The back gable of our house faces due north. In the middle of the night, if I look out of the window next to my bed and track upward in a straight line from the highest branches of the fig tree at the top of the little hill in front of me, I see Polaris, the

North Star. The bottom arms of Ursa Major reach out toward her on one side, and on the other the receptive "W" of Cassiopeia faces her in irregular, branch-like asymmetry. Night after night, when I look up, there is Polaris. By early morning all the other stars in the northern sky have rotated in an arc from east to west, but not Polaris. Polaris is the one point in the northern night sky that does not move. She is always in the same place.

In the early hours of the morning on the second night of my vision quest, I was suddenly awakened by the sound of earth moving just inches from my head. I sat bolt upright and turned around to face whatever it was. All was silent. I turned in the direction of the sound. On the small, bare hill that bordered the edge of my site, in the dim moonlight, I saw a giant toad sitting motionless, its body still partially buried in the ground. Maybe he had smelled the moisture from the recent rain and decided to come out of hibernation. After a little while I heard him scurry off into the brush. Then all was quiet again.

I sat up to focus on my prayer. I knelt before the altar in the corner, struck a match, and burned some dried white sage. I smudged myself down and then I smudged the sacred pipe. I picked it up and stooped forward, holding the pipe bowl to my heart and the stem to my forehead, almost touching the ground. As I began to pray for the future generations, I noticed that I was feeling disconnected from my prayer. There was something abstract about the words "future generations" that felt far removed from my own experience. I turned my prayers to the reality of the ripening life in my daughter Mary-Anna's belly. Pictures came into my mind: a clear-cut forest, a scraped bare mountaintop, parched broken earth, and a shot wolf, his hindquarters all bloodied, looking straight at the photographer with his tongue out and an open, smiling face. Questions came: "Is there even going to be a future for the unborn to come into? And what can I do about this?" For some time, I knelt there holding these questions as I continued to pray and sing.

I stood up. Before me there was a great scrub oak. From its silhouette, I could count sixteen separate boughs descending to its single base. I imagined clasping one of the boughs and pressing it hard against my aching heart. I closed my eyes. The ache became a yearning for the welfare of the future ones. I opened my eyes. The splayed branches of the oak looked even blacker now against the dark Prussian-blue sky. Suddenly I noticed the stars, shining through the mottled canopy of black. My gaze continued upward over my head. The sky was full of the brightest stars I had ever seen. As my eyes were touched by light from the distant past, words came: "We are already here."

Silently I asked, "Given that you're already here, what can I do for you now? What can I do now so that you future ones will be born into a world as beautiful as this one; this world surrounding me on this altar, with the mountains, the sages, the meadows, the flowers coming out after the rains, the grasses, the clouds, the birds, the oaks?"

Then, directly above my head, and straight over the red, northern flag, I noticed a small bright star standing alone that I immediately recognized. Its name flashed into my mind—but not as the North Star, not as Polaris, but as *bodhichitta*, a word and a concept I had been introduced to by Joanna Macy. I knew that I was being given an answer to my question. I began to pray, "May I walk beautifully on the Earth so that they may walk beautifully on the Earth. May I do what I can do to make this world a better place for the future ones. May everyone who lives now and in the future, know that they are beloved of the Earth."

The word *bodhichitta* is made up of two Sanskrit words: *bodhi*, meaning "awakened" and, *chitta*, meaning "heart-mind." Joanna speaks of how, "in the Buddhist tradition, *bodhichitta* is seen as something very precious, something to treasure and protect. We can think of it as a flame in our hearts and minds that guides us and shines through our actions."[1] *Bodhichitta* describes a particular intention and motivation. As she puts it, "*Bodhichitta* is the overarching yearning for the welfare of all beings." *Bodhichitta* is an ember that each of us carries in our hearts, which in the right conditions blazes into being.

Like the North Star, *bodhichitta* is always there to come back to. It reorients and situates us in a stream of interdependence that transforms suffering—that of others and our own. When our personal welfare is our primary concern, we reinforce our sense of separateness and disconnection. This feeds our fear and insecurity, and intensifies our suffering. When we make the well-being of others our primary concern, it strengthens our experience of interconnectedness and of being part of something greater. This soothes our fear and brings us into healing.

I have heard his Holiness the Dalai Lama say that he begins his day at 3:00 a.m. with practices to cultivate bodhichitta. When he was asked, "What keeps you from being overwhelmed when you see what is happening in Tibet and to your fellow countrymen?" he replied: "I trust in the sincerity of my heart's intentions." And when he was asked, "During the course of your life, what have been your greatest lessons?" he replied, "Mostly *bodhichitta*, altruism. It has helped a lot. In some ways, you could say *bodhichitta* has made me into a new person, a new man. I am still progressing. Trying. It gives you inner strength, courage, and it is easier to accept situations."[2]

Bodhichitta is the altruistic intention that fuels compassionate action. *Bodhichitta* is the North Star to guide us in uncertain times. *Bodhichitta* is a powerful medicine that makes it possible to live with pain.

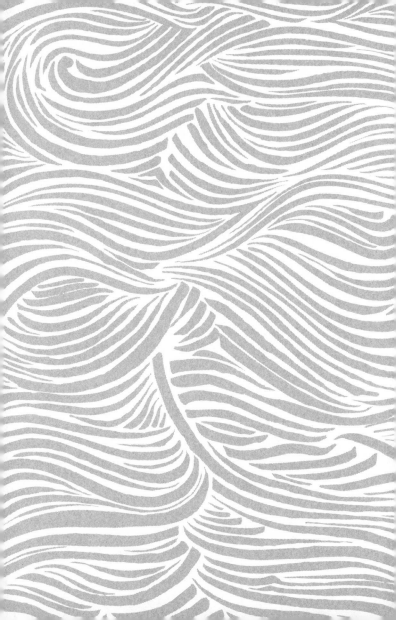

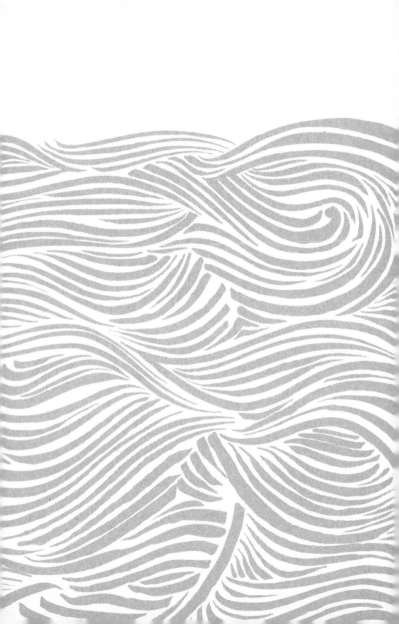

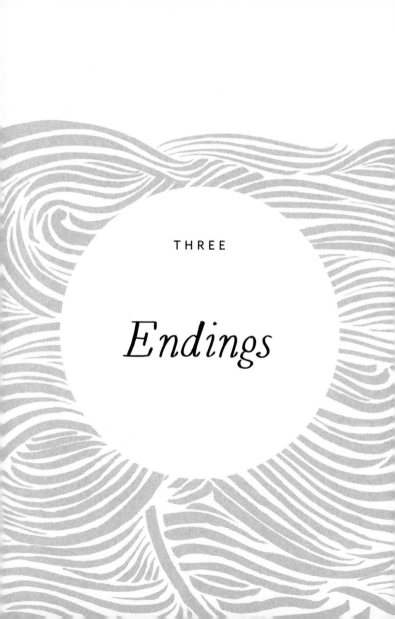

THREE

Endings

MONDAY EVENING, JUNE

Last night I woke up full of concerns for Ben, my patient. I realized that despite everything we had done, he was getting weaker and there was nothing that I or anyone else could do to prevent this. I sat up on the side of my bed and looked out the window. The sky was so bright from the full moon that at first I did not see any stars. Then I looked above the fig tree and there it was, Polaris, the North Star. Immediately, I saw Ben's face: so young, so emaciated, so wanting to hope, so undemanding. Silently, and thinking of Ben, I recited a *bodhichitta* prayer: "May all beings be happy, may all beings be safe, may all beings everywhere be free, and may I become all that I need to become to best enable this to happen."

As I prayed, I felt the emotional resonance of the words. When I had finished, I continued to sit there looking at the star. I noticed that something about my feelings had changed. Where there had been worry and a sense of failure, there was sadness, affection, and deep appreciation for this courageous young man.

Ben never made it home. He never got to see his granddad again. Instead he came straight to the inpatient hospice because he was so weak and still in so much pain. During the first couple of weeks in the hospice he did well. It seemed as if he saw this move as a new beginning and a new opportunity, and that he wanted to do what he could to make the most of it. His pain settled down, and with the help of a friend who was a nutritionist, he started on a diet of organic fruits, vegetables, and juices. Many people, caregivers as well as family, commented on a change they noticed in Ben. Whereas before he had kept his room darkened, now it was bright and filled with sunlight. He said he felt well and, having previously not wanted visitors, he now welcomed family and friends. He took time each day to sit out on the patio to feel the warm air and listen to the running water of the water fountain, and watch the birds in the coastal oaks. His thirty-first birthday was on May 30. It was also his mother's birthday, and happened to be the day of his grandfather's funeral. Ben went to the funeral and insisted on walking from the car to his place in the church. The following day he told me how important it was for him to have been able to do this and to see some of his favorite uncles and aunts.

Four weeks after his admission to hospice, Ben's situation was looking very different. He had lost a lot of weight in the past couple of weeks and his pain was worsening. We had adjusted his pain medication and this had helped, but he was now sleeping more due to the increased sedation and his weakening body. When I saw him early in the afternoon, he was curled up in his bed asleep. The room was once again darkened. Juanita, his mother, was at his bedside. Ben looked shrunken and very much weaker than when I had last seen him. When I sat by his bedside and gently called his name, he opened his eyes and said "Hello, Doctor Kearney." Then he closed his eyes again. I told him I would be back later to see how he was doing. As I left, Juanita followed me out into the corridor. I suggested we sit and talk in the nearby family room.

Juanita said, "I've been praying for a miracle but I can see what's happening with his body. I sat with my father when he was dying. He fought it for so long. At the end I was able to say to him, 'It's okay to go now.' I know that this is what's happening for Ben, but I can't say to my son, 'It's okay to go …' Because it's not. I don't know what to say to him." She began to cry. I too felt at a loss and for a while we just sat there together in silence. Then I said, "I don't know what to say either, Juanita. Maybe it's not so much about words anymore. Maybe it's just about being with him now. Your presence says it all."

When I came back later in the afternoon, Ben seemed to be more deeply asleep. I pulled over a chair and sat at the opposite side of the bed from Juanita. Ben looked so frail, peaceful, and comfortable lying there. His breathing was smooth and easy. After a little while I said, "Ben, it's okay to sleep. You sleep now, my friend, as much as you like…. Your granddad is close by…. I'll look in tomorrow." Without opening his eyes, he said, "Thank you." I put my hand on his very thin, tattooed arm and left the room. As I left the hospice house, an unexpected gentle rain was falling.

Later that evening as I sit in the dark in the sweat lodge, I think of Ben and Juanita. I am filled with sadness that this beautiful young life that is just beginning is coming to an end. Wolf asks, "Does anyone have a prayer that needs to be spoken out loud?"

"*For all my relations!*" I answer.

"Yes, relative," Wolf replies.

I pray for Ben, that he be free of suffering, that he find healing, that he find his way. And I pray for Juanita, for a blessing on her heart and that she too may be free of suffering and find the healing she needs.

As Lisa begins to sing and others join in, I sit back and drop deeper into the dark. It's hot now and the lodge is filled with the breath of the stone people. My eyes are closed and sweat is pouring down my face like tears and falling onto the earth by my feet. I see the nest in the stream. As the water flows, it begins to turn, slowly, sun-wise, and as it does, something at its black core begins to glow—an ember, an intensity, a star—and filaments of light flicker out in all directions. I pray that this light touches Ben and Juanita, and all who suffer, nearby and far away, those I know and those I don't know.

LESSONS FROM NATURE

As a child, I loved nature but always from a distance and on my terms. Then, with the tragic drowning of the girls in the river by our home, I was swept into the realization that nature has a pulse and agency of her own. This is a lesson I have been taught again and again since then as other-than-human nature has come toward me. As I lay on the Earth in my grief, she came toward me as the robin. As I came to the Earth in my curiosity, she approached me as the wolf on the road in Yellowstone. As I walked the land near our home with gratitude and respect, she revealed her beauty as junco, as grandfather rock, as grandmother white sage, as red-tailed hawk, and as morning light on the grasses. As I returned to the Earth with my heart's deepest question, the ladybug nation reminded me that I too belong. When I asked the Earth how I could come back into right relations with the rest of nature, she led me into a dance with the Tree Nation, and reminded me that I too have roots. Nature is no longer something I love from a distance but who I am in my deepest identity.

Nature teaches me that connection awakens *bodhichitta*, which in turn awakens connection. A recurring theme in the teachings I have received from nature is that the more deeply connected I am to another, the more I care about that person; and that the more I care, the more I long to act, to do what I can to relieve that person's suffering, and the suffering of others. The better I got to know Ben, the more I wanted to visit and spend time with him and do what I could to help him, even when this meant walking into a room thick with grief. But it did not end there. Doing what I could to help Ben did not satisfy my yearning to relieve suffering. On the contrary, it deepened that yearning, while at the same time sustaining and empowering me to move toward the next person in pain, and the next.

So too, as I grow closer to the California towhee couple I meet by the corner every morning and as I have become more aware of the complex yet delicate ecosystem they inhabit, the more concerned I have become about their welfare. Again, it does not stop there. I notice that this increases my sensitivity to environmental concerns further afield, and the impact these changes will have for the future generations.

I imagine myself standing at the side of the creek, watching the clear, silent water flowing through the loose and open weave of the nest. The nest in the stream teaches me how to be with my pain. It teaches me that what really matters is setting my intention, being willing to suffer my suffering, and choosing to surrender. For the sake of all beings, I can let the pain in, allow myself to feel it, and then, rather than holding onto it, I can let it go. But even then, there is a further letting go; I can let the pain go to some deeper stream that is always flowing through, some bigger story in which I am a participant and not the author. Finally, the nest in the stream teaches me more than a way of being with pain; it offers a way of being in the world.

"So, how can I be in the world?" I ask.

"Lightly, lightly, lightly," the nest in the stream replies.

A STORY ENDS

For some days now, Ben has been right on the cusp of life and death. In a deep and comfortable sleep, his body has been gently preparing him to die. Juanita is by his side night and day. She is ready to let him go now. She has been telling him this and that his grandfather is waiting for him. Today she had left for a little while but was called back by the nurses who had noticed a change in his breathing.

Endings

It's late that afternoon and I am about to leave to go home. I am planning to go into the sweat lodge later this evening. I decide to go back and look in on Ben one last time. As I go into the room, Juanita is sitting at the far side of the bed holding his hand. I pull over a chair on the other side and take Ben's left hand in mine. It's cold. I watch his face. He is not breathing. After perhaps half a minute his chest rises with a gasp, and then another, and another. "He's very close," I say. "It may be just a matter of hours." I gently squeeze Ben's hand and silently say my goodbye. I stand. I say to Juanita, "I need to go now. I leave him with you. There's someone just outside the door. Please call if you have any concerns or worries... It's good that you're here."

Ben is on my mind as I arrive at the fireplace. In the lodge, I wait for the third round, which is dedicated to the grandfather in the west. In this round, we especially remember those who are near the West Gate, those who are close to death and those who have already passed over. As Wolf finishes a song, there is silence. I say, *"For all my relations!"* He replies, "Yes, relative."

I pray for Ben, who is so ready, who is so close, that he may pass safely and peacefully. I pray for Juanita, who is also ready now, that she may see him leave this world in gentleness and beauty. Wolf says he is now going to sing a song he rarely sings in the lodge. It's a song for one who, like Ben, is close to the West Gate and about to cross over.

Alone, and without a drumbeat, Wolf begins to sing. The

song is stark and strong and tender. As he sings, he pours water onto the stones. My eyes are closed tight as the breath of the stone people rises and fills the lodge. In the dark within the dark I find myself in Ben's room, looking down on him from above. Juanita is there bent forward, head down on the bed in exhaustion, or grief, or both. Ben's face is as it was that afternoon. His eyes are sunken and closed. He looks like a monk in prayer in an El Greco painting. Then he opens his eyes. Juanita does not seem to notice as he gets out of bed, pauses, and leaning toward her, kisses her on the back of her head. He walks around the foot of the bed to the French doors that lead to the patio. He opens them wide and steps through. In the night sky, there's a young moon and there are stars in the oak trees. His grandfather is there too. Waiting.

As I sit there in the break before the third and final round, I realize that I have become attached to a particular outcome. I am ready for Ben to pass. I think, "Maybe he crossed over just now, as Wolf sang his song. Maybe this is what I was seeing." And then I think, "And maybe not... What's happening now is between Ben and the Great Mystery." And I find that I am able to let go a little. Ben will move on when the time is right—and, ultimately, that is not my business.

At the end of the ceremony, after Lisa finishes a song of gratitude, Wolf says, "May the peace at the heart of these stones penetrate us, and when we leave this lodge, may we be an encouragement to others, maybe in ways we don't even understand, and not feed the discouragement that's out there." He adds, "The only way to keep a blessing is to give it away." Then he says, "All together now!"

"For all my relations!" we cry out with one voice.

"Raise the flap!" Wolf calls, and cold air rushes in.

The next morning, I go in early to see Ben. Juanita is there. She has spent the night with him. She is planning to go home soon for a few hours. She has decided to give Ben more space. "He loved being on his own when he was well. Maybe that's what he needs now too." I say my sense is that he is right on the threshold and that he is crossing over and coming back. She says, "Yes, I sense that too." I tell her that I have something I want to share with her. I describe how I prayed for Ben the night before at a Native American sweat lodge ceremony. I describe Wolf's song and what I had seen happening in my mind's eye. When I finished, she is silent for a little while. Then she says, "Yesterday afternoon we pushed Ben's bed out onto the patio. It was so beautiful out there. There was birdsong and the sounds of running water...."

* * *

Throughout my working life, I have had mixed feelings about

my chosen profession. On many occasions, I have thought about leaving medicine to follow my passion in another direction, whether this was English literature, making movies, depth psychology, or spiritual direction. However, again and again, life circumstances have gently nudged me back into my career as a doctor. The same dynamic surfaced in the journey I have talked about here. Repeatedly I have asked myself, and with growing frustration, what all this signifies. Does it mean that I need to leave medicine to walk more deeply on the Red Road? Or become a full-time teacher of Joanna Macy's Work that Reconnects? Or find a way to teach deep nature connection practices with Jon Young and his team? Again and again I seemed to hear the answer, "No, that's not it."

On the second morning of Sun Dance, as I was joining in the dance with the other supporters from the edge of the arbor, a question came to mind. I had come all this way; I had come to the outer circle of the arbor, and I was standing there watching as a new dancer was being led to the buffalo robe on the ground to be "pierced up" so he could be attached to the Tree of Life. I did not feel any desire to do this. At that moment I knew with certainty that this is not something I would ever do.

I had immediately started to doubt myself. What was happening here? Was I hitting a cultural glass wall? Was this, I asked myself, as far as I, a "paleface," could go on the Red Road? Was this what D. H. Lawrence meant when he said, "We

[Europeans] cannot cluster at the drum anymore?"[1] Yet, I told myself, this did not seem to be true, firstly because of my own experience up until then, and secondly, because when I looked into the arbor, I saw that a number of the pierced Sun Dancers were at least as white as I am. Or, I wondered, was it simply because I was too afraid to step beyond my comfort zone into the unknown? I remember feeling confused as I walked up the hill to camp that evening.

That night I had the following dream: Radhule and I were considering buying a house in London from a young couple, a husband and wife who had one child. There were spacious open-plan rooms and big windows with lots of light. I walked up to one of the windows and looked outside. It was like the west of Ireland. There was a lake going off into the distance, with hills ascending into the mist on either side. The water on the lake was very calm. All around the house the ground was uneven and grassy, and there were old trees, mostly oaks, and rocks coming right up to the house. In the distance, I could see a city skyline. There were skyscrapers on the horizon. I realized that this was a house in the wilderness in the city! Then I noticed that the dining room had a grass floor. There was lots of light coming in and I thought, "I could grow vegetables inside as well as outside under the old oaks and among the rocks, and living here would allow us to be closer to our families!" I awoke with a sense of clarity. I knew in a way I did not understand that I had received an answer to the questions I had been asking the day before.

As I joined the other supporters in the arbor on the final day of Sun Dance, I was filled with feelings of gratitude for Wolf and Lisa and all the teachings I had received from them, and for this beautiful ceremony of which I was so privileged to be a part. Then a wave of gratitude for my other teachers swept through me—for John Moriarty, for Joanna Macy, and for Jon Young. I saw how I had been led from one to the other of these teachers over the years in a widening spiral of instruction and understanding, and how each had included the others' wisdom while bringing in something unique and different of their own. Once again, I knew that I had come as far as I could with each of these teachers. But now I saw it differently. It was not that I was too scared to commit to any one of these paths. I saw that "How can I leave medicine to do what I am really being called to do?" was in fact the wrong question. I saw how the teachings I had received were like the interweaving twigs and branches of the nest in the stream. I remembered the wilderness dream house in the city. And I knew that all these teachings would be in my heart as I took my next step forward.

There is an old Irish story of a famous warrior called Bran Mac Feabhail. In John Moriarty's account,[2] we hear of how Bran had a vision one night of a silver branch that hovered, shimmering in the dark before him. He felt deeply unsettled by this and returned to his room. There he found a beautiful woman who said she came from the Otherworld. In song, she described this Otherworld and invited Bran to come and visit her there. The next day he set out with three boats. Despite Bran's coaxing, the crew made little progress against the furious headwinds. Then Bran saw something that caused him to fall silent. Coming toward him through the storm was Manannan, the god of the sea, in a chariot drawn by four great white horses. Manannan looked Bran straight in the eye.

"What do you see when you look out there?" he asked.

"I see gray waves," Bran replied.

"Here's what I see," Manannan said, and he began to sing.

His descriptions of what he saw were identical to what the beautiful woman had said about the Otherworld. As Bran listened, understanding grew in him and he broke his silence. He called to his captains to turn around the boats and head for home. As he watched the green mountains on the horizon grow larger, he realized that he had just been gifted with something priceless that he could not put into words. His thoughts were interrupted by the crunch of the boat's prow on the pebble beach. He looked up. Standing there in front of him on the shore of Ireland was the beautiful woman. In the air beside her was the singing silver branch.

It was only when Bran stepped off the boat onto the land and looked around that he understood where he was. He had arrived in the Otherworld, and yet it was the same world he had left early that same morning. On the outside nothing was different, and yet nothing was the same. Something fundamental had changed. He realized then what had happened. What he had been gifted with was another way of seeing—what John Moriarty calls "silver branch perception;" a way of seeing that this world, and not some other world, is paradise.

I, like Bran, supposed that I was being called to another world. Instead, I find that at the end of this journey I have come back to the same world I thought I had left behind. In my day job, I continue to work as a palliative care doctor, doing what I can to treat my patients' pain. And I have noticed something else. I am no longer burnt out. Where the inner ground was dry and crisp and desperately thirsty, there is now the sound of running water. My occupation, what I do in the world, is no longer an issue. This journey was not leading up to a career change after all, but to an inner dissolution; a melting way of encrusted and encrusting ways of being, and seeing, and acting.

As a doctor, while I continue to do what I can to alleviate pain and suffering, I do so now knowing that in tending the microcosm, I am tending the macrocosm; in caring for the part, I am caring for the whole. There is no gap between doing all I can to relieve Ben's pain, and being with him as he slowly realizes that he is not going to get better, and doing what I can to heal our ailing world.

Endings

* * *

It's early morning and I have come out onto the south-facing patio of our home. I have just heard from the hospice that Ben passed away at 12:30 a.m., quietly, peacefully, and on his own. Late yesterday afternoon his older brother, whom he had not seen for some time, had arrived from up north. He and Juanita and her sister had stayed with Ben through the evening and then had gone home to get some sleep.

I close my eyes and see Ben breathing out, and out, and out. I watch him continuing to breathe out beyond the end of the exhale, letting go, letting go, letting go. He comes to a pause. I wait. And wait. This time his body does not breathe again. He has slipped away like an otter beneath the water's surface, without so much as a ripple. In the end, his was such a gentle dying.

There are still many stars in the sky. I imagine how each star could be an ancestor, or a future being, or one of the countless trillions of living beings alive on this planet today. The sky is full of all my relations. It's brightening in the east. I think of how, as the dawn rises and light comes into the sky, the stars will begin to fade until eventually they are all gone and there is only the brightness of the sky.

I too have slipped back beneath the surface of my life. In my everyday circumstances, I have returned to where I began. I think of those lines of T. S. Eliot: "And the end of all our exploring/ Will be to arrive where we started/ And know the place for the first time."[3] Nothing has changed and yet everything is different.

As I stood with everyone else at the edge of the arbor on the last day of Sun Dance, an image came to me. I saw three figures. To the left was a great old oak, rooted deep, with a thick trunk and branches that were full of dark green foliage reaching out in graceful irregularity in all directions. I was standing next to it. The lower part of my body was a red-brown tree trunk and I too was rooted in the Earth. My right arm was stretched out and intertwined with a branch of the oak. My left hand was reaching upward, holding the outstretched hand of a person who was floating with legs like helium balloons up in the air.

Perhaps connection is not something we *do* but a process; a state of being and a way of life. Perhaps connection is, ultimately, who we are.

"At the end of the day, does any of this make a blind bit of difference?" the cynic in me asks.

"I don't know," some other voice within replies, "but I feel it does."

When I got out of bed this morning, my heart ached. As I walked down the hill with the dogs, I was glad to see the towhees were there by the side of the road. A scrub jay looped in and lingered on the branch of a young oak before continuing across the road. There were white blossoms with blood-red cups lying scattered on the ground. As I approached the corner, the bells of Santa Barbara Mission rang. I could smell newly laid mulch nearby. It's as though all my senses are more awake these days.

I know that the ache in my heart is not about me. It's about Bill, another young patient of mine who is dying in a fog of confusion, with anguished parents who have just arrived from New Zealand. It's about the drowned little boy Alan Kurdi lying face down on a Turkish beach, who could be my grandson Elliot. It's about the melting icecaps and the vanishing rainforests. It's about all my relations. It is not as though I did not have these feelings before. I did, but they were blunted and tame. Now they are unfiltered and raw.

INTO THE DEEPER STREAM

Some refer to synchronicities as "miracles." Zen teacher Suzuki Roshi writes, "Gaining enlightenment is an accident. Practice makes us accident-prone."[1] We all know that we cannot make miracles happen, much as we might want to. But, as I have already said, this does not mean that there is nothing we can do to make it more likely that such events will occur.

I have had some extraordinary teachers during these past fifteen years whose instructions have taught me how to come into deep connection with nature and how to be with my pain. A number of practices based on what I have learned from my teachers, and from the experiences I have shared in my stories, have become part of my daily routine. These make me more "accident-prone."

I end this book by describing my daily practices to share what helps me to come into deep connection and to a peaceful way of being with my pain. While these practices work for me, I do not wish to imply that they will work for everyone. While some readers will find them helpful, others will not. Feel free to try them, and take what works and discard what doesn't. What matters is that we each have our own ways of coming regularly and reliably into deep connection with other-than-human nature, with others, and with ourselves; it matters that we are willing to feel whatever pain we are feeling; and it matters that we know we can release our pain to the flowing through of the deeper stream for the sake of all beings.

* * *

In the middle of the night, if I look out of our bedroom window, I see the North Star. I touch my hand to my heart, and say a prayer. I may do this in a variety of possible ways. For example, I might say (to myself), *"For all my relations!"* or, "May all beings be happy!"

* * *

Each morning, before leaving for work, I practice mindfulness of breathing meditation. I have deepened in my love of this practice and again and again am amazed to see how the simple act of paying attention to and becoming one with the sensations of breathing can, even in the most turbulent of times, bring me into bright, still, clear awareness. I have also come to value mindfulness of breathing as a practice of "inner nature connection." In attending to and merging my awareness with the sensations of breathing, I am remembering the effortless, reciprocal exchange between my body and all that breathes.

* * *

If I have time in the morning, I may continue from mindfulness of breathing to a practice that merges elements of Joanna Macy's "Breathing through Meditation"[2] with my own experience of the nest in the stream. Here, having first taken time to come into the sensations of the body's breathing, I shift the focus of my awareness to the center of my chest in the area of my heart and notice whatever sensations are there. More specifically, I attend to whatever sensations of pain are in my heart, perhaps an ache, or a tightness, or a turbulence that has been lingering since the phone call I took about a patient during the night, and I allow my awareness to drop into these sensations for just a few moments; to feel whatever it is I am feeling in my heart. Then, letting this be, I bring my attention back to the sensations of breath, as it flows in with the inhale, and as it is flows through with the exhale.

I picture the breath as a breathstream that flows in with the inhale, and down through my chest with the exhale. I sense the sensations of the breath stream, as it flows in and as it flows through. I pay particular attention to the sensations of the exhale, as the breathstream washes around and through the nest of my heart, carrying the pain in its flow. I remind myself that the breathstream is flowing through without my volition. I end by consciously releasing the energy of the pain or whatever feelings are in my heart to the great flow of life, for the sake of all beings.

* * *

Occasionally I like to alternate my breathing through the heart practice with a gratitude practice. From my Native American teachers, I have learned about the value of gratitude as a form of prayer. Wolf teaches that gratitude is not a "should." He says that practicing gratitude means noticing what we are already grateful for and allowing ourselves to be with the felt-sense of this in our body. I have noticed that this practice softens and opens my heart.

I learned a gratitude practice called "Orderly Fashion Prayer" from Jon Young, who was taught it by Lakota elder Gilbert Walking Bull,[3] and I like to combine this with an honoring of the four directions. I begin by turning (in my mind's eye) to the east and remembering what gives my life its greatest meaning. I notice whatever feelings of gratitude rise up in my heart as I do this, and for just a few moments, I allow myself to linger with the felt-sense of this.

Next, having turned toward the south, I give thanks for creation. As I do this, I recall any encounters with other-than-human nature that I have been touched by in the past twenty-four hours. For example, this morning I remembered how yesterday, as I left the parking lot at work, a dark-eyed junco had hopped from the under the shrubs onto the pavement just a few feet in front of me. I had paused for a few moments and watched him as he fed from the sidewalk, before stepping around him. He was still feeding when I looked back in his direction. As

I remember this, I notice a gentle upsurge of joy in my heart. I allow my awareness to drop into how this feels in my body, and for just a few breaths, allow myself to rest in this simple happiness.

Next, as I turn toward the west, I look toward my fellow humans, my loved ones, my patients, my teachers, those who are living and those who have already passed on. I notice whoever comes to mind as I do this. I picture this person as if they are standing before me. I allow our eyes to meet and notice whatever feelings of gratitude arise in my heart. Once again, I linger with my feelings of gratitude that this individual is part of my life, and I pray a blessing on her or him.

Finally, I turn toward the north and give thanks for my own life; for being alive in the world at this time, and for the blessings I receive in such abundance. I rest for just a few moments in how this feels in my body. I may end with the short prayer, "My heart is yours, Grandmother, Grandfather, my heart is yours; for the people, for all the people."

* * *

I practice nature connection many times during the day, for example, while walking the dogs to the corner of the street where we live and back each morning, or when I take them on their daily late afternoon walk to a small oak forest by a creek.

Occasionally I stop and give my full sensory awareness to what I am hearing, seeing, touching, smelling, or even tasting. For example, if I notice birdsong, I may close my eyes and bring my full attention to what I am hearing. Rather than trying to analyze the sounds, I openly receive them, and then, with the exhale, let my awareness drop down into the felt-sense experiencing of them. If I find my attention has been carried away by thoughts or worries, as soon as I notice this, I relax, let go of the thought or the worry, and allow my awareness to fall back into the body and the sensation I am experiencing.

As I walk from the parking lot to the palliative care office by the long route, sun-wise around the hospital rather than through it, I pay attention to the young live oaks that line the roadway. I sometimes sing the sweat lodge song of welcome for the stone people as I walk and notice the clouds, or the breeze, or linger for a moment in the cool of the shade before stepping again into the white heat of midday.

* * *

As I enter the palliative care office, or the hospice, or the hospital, or the room of a patient, or as I put my hand on the door handle on my way into a meeting, I pause to remember that there are elements in what I am about to encounter that are beyond me. I may repeat the prayer, "My heart is yours, Grandmother, Grandfather, my heart is yours; for the people, for all the people."

More and more I have come to rely on the breathing through the heart practice to get me through my working day. If I am feeling upset or overwhelmed, as I was yesterday listening to a patient's young wife, who was weeping as she spoke about her utter helplessness in the face of her husband's awful suffering, I will find the earliest opportunity I can to take a short "time out." If possible, I try to find a quiet corner of the hospital, or a window where I can stand and look out at the trees for a few moments, or better still, I step outside into a patch of shade in the fresh air for a little while. I then go through a four-step practice of mindfully breathing through my pain. Firstly, I notice and sense the sensations of breathing. Next I notice whatever pain is in my heart and allow myself to feel this. Then, I return to the sensations of the breath, paying special attention to the exhale, feeling how it moves through my body. Finally, I consciously release my pain to the next exhale, and the next, surrendering all to the effortless flow. This does not take long, just minute or so, but it makes a big difference to how I feel and how I am as I continue through my day.

Endings

* * *

As often as I can, I go to what Jon Young calls a "sit spot,"[4] my special place in nature to which I return regularly to spend some time. I have a number of sit spots. The one I use most is in my own backyard. I also have one in a park about five minutes' walk from the hospital where I can occasionally escape for a five-to ten-minute sit. These are places I have become familiar with from the simple acts of visiting, hanging out, and paying attention with respect to all aspects of what is going on there. It is my hope that these places have become familiar with me too.

I notice the behavior of birds and other creatures, as well as plants, and rocks, and other features of the landscape, such as the temperature, the light and shade, the wind, and the moisture in the earth, or the lack of it. When I return to the hospital after even a very short visit to my sit spot close by, I feel refreshed and well and as though I am an ambassador for what poet E. E. Cummings calls, "The leaping greenly spirit of things."[5]

* * *

Most Monday evenings, having finished at the hospital and stopped off briefly at home, I meet up with some friends to carpool and drive an hour south to the weekly sweat lodge ceremony offered by Wolf and Lisa. Even if I am tired and stressed at the end of the working day, as I often am, I inevitably make this journey with a growing sense of excitement and gratitude to have such an opportunity of prayer and community just down the road. I enjoy sitting and chatting with friends before the lodge begins as we gather in a circle around the sacred fire. I often enter the lodge with pain and sadness for patients in my care. Sometimes I pray out loud. More often I pray for them silently. In the ceremony, whatever pain I am experiencing merges with the medicines of the sacred herbs, the breath of the stone people, the singing, sometimes the smoke of the sacred pipe, and as the sweat flows down my body and onto the ground, I feel lighter and cleaner.

By the time I return home from the sweat lodge, it's late and my beloved wife is sound asleep. I know that in just a few hours I will be getting up for the weekly interdisciplinary team meeting at the hospice. I pause and look out the north-facing window beside my bed. There is that bright star all on its own, straight above the top branches of the fig tree. Silently, I say to myself, *"For all my relations!"*

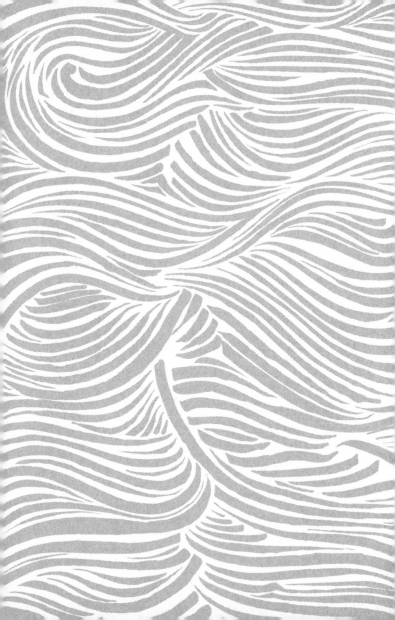

NOTES

Epigraph from Rainer Maria Rilke, *Rilke's Book of Hours: Love Poems to God*, trans. Anita Barrows and Joanna Macy (New York: Riverhead, 2005), 171.

A SEARCH FOR HEALING

1. Rainer Maria Rilke, *Rilke's Book of Hours: Love Poems to God*, trans. Anita Barrows and Joanna Macy (New York: Riverhead, 2005), 45.
2. William Wordsworth, "Intimations of Immortality from Recollections of Early Childhood," *Poems of Wordsworth* (London: Macmillan St Martin's Press), 203.
3. To read more about Jean Vanier, see Jean Vanier, https://en.wikipedia.org/wiki/Jean_Vanier.
4. Cicely Saunders, *The Management of Terminal Malignant Disease* (London: Edward Arnold, 1978), 194.
5. Carl Gustav Jung, letter of July 10, 1946, in C.G. Jung, *Letters 1: 1906–1950*, 433.
6. Károly Kerényi, Asklepios: *Archetypal Image of the Physician's Existence* (New York: Bollingen Foundation, 1959), 25-26.
7. G.E.R. Lloyd (ed.), *Hippocratic Writings* (London: Penguin Classics, 1978), 39.
8. Brian Doyle, *The Wet Engine: Exploring the Mad Wild Miracle of the Heart* (Brewster: Massachusetts, 2005)
9. Nicholas Black Elk, *Black Elk Speaks: Being the Story of a Holy Man of the Oglala Sioux*, as told through John G. Neihart (Lincoln: University of Nebraska Press, 1979).
10. Joanna Macy, *Mutual Causality in Buddhism and General Systems Theory* (Albany: State University of New York Press, 1991).
11. Alan Wallace, *30 Guided Meditations: Short Introductory Meditation* (Santa Barbara: Santa Barbara Institute for Consciousness Studies).

12. Robert Bly, *The Kabir Book: Forty-Four of the Ecstatic Poems of Kabir* (Boston: Beacon Press, 1977), 52.

13. Joanna Macy, *Coming Back to Life: The Updated Guide to "The Work that Reconnects"* (Gabriola Island, British Columbia, Canada: New Society Publishers, 2014).

RELATING TO PAIN

1. Coleman Barks, trans., "Childhood Friends," *The Essential Rumi* (San Francisco: Harper Collins, 1996), 142.

2. Michael Kearney et al., Self-care of physicians caring for patients at the end-of-life: "Being connected... a key to my survival," *The Journal of the American Medical Association* 301, 11 (March 18, 2009): 1155-1164.

SEVEN STORIES OF NATURE CONNECTION

1. Jon Young, Elle Hass, Evan McGown, *Coyote's Guide to Connecting with Nature* (Santa Cruz, California: OWLink Media, 2010).

2. Thich Nhat Hahn, *Interbeing: Fourteen Precepts for Engaged Buddhism* (Berkeley, California: Parallax Press, 1987).

FIRST: COLMAN'S WELL

1. R. S. Thomas, from "Here," *Collected Poems 1945–1990* (London: Phoenix Giants, 1993), 120.

2. Rainer Maria Rilke, *The Selected Poetry of Rainer Maria Rilke*, trans. Stephen Mitchell (New York: Vintage International, 1989), 135.

THIRD: THE LAND

1. Mary Oliver, *New and Selected Poems* (Boston: Beacon Press, 1992).
2. John Moriarty, *One Evening in Eden: Tridium Sacrum*, Vol. 2, Audio CD set (Dublin: Sli no Firinne Foundation, The Lilliput Press, 2007).
3. Jon Young, *What the Robin Knows: How Birds Reveal the Secrets of the Natural World* (Boston: Houghton Mifflin Harcourt, 2012), xxv.
4. Mary Oliver, *Winter Hours* (Boston: Houghton Mifflin), 96-97.
5. Young, *What the Robin Knows: How Birds Reveal the Secrets of the Natural World*, 63-64, 175.

FOURTH: THE NEST IN THE STREAM

1. John Moriarty, *One Evening in Eden: Eden*, Vol. 2, Audio CD set (Dublin: Sli no Firinne Foundation, The Lilliput Press, 2007).
2. Bernie Glassman: http://zenpeacemakers.org/bernie-glassman/
3. Eugene Gendlin, *Focusing* (New York: Bantam New Age Books, Random House, 1982).
4. Carl Gustav Jung, cited in P. W. Martin, *An Experiment in Depth: A Study of the Work of Jung*, Eliot, and Toynbee (London: Routledge & Kegan Paul, 1987).

SIXTH: THE TREE OF LIFE

1. Friedrich Nietzsche, *Maxims and Arrows 12 from Twilight of the Idols, or, How to Philosophize with a Hammer*, originally published as *Götzen-Dämmerung, oder, Wie man mit dem Hammer philosophirt*, 1888, quoted in Viktor Frankl, *Man's Search for Meaning* 1992 Edition (Boston: Beacon Press, 1992).

SEVENTH: POLARIS

1. Joanna Macy, *Active Hope: How to Face the Mess We're in without Going Crazy* (Novato, California: New World Library, 2012), 233.
2. His Holiness the Dalai Lama: https://www.dalailama.com/the-dalai-lama/biography-and-daily-life/questions-answers.

A STORY ENDS

1. D.H. Lawrence, *Mornings in Mexico and Other Essays,* ed., Virginia Crosswhite Hyde; essay, *Indians and an Englishman,* (Cambridge: Cambridge University Press, 2014), 120.
2. John Moriarty, *What the Curlew Said: Nostos Continued,* (Dublin: The Lilliput Press, 2007), 111-112.
3. T.S. Eliot, "Little Gidding," *The Four Quartets* (Boston & New York: Mariner Books, Houghton Mifflin Harcourt, 1971), 59.

INTO THE DEEPER STREAM

1. Shunryu Suzuki Roshi, cited in Jack Kornfield, *After the Ecstasy the Laundry: How the Heart Grows Wise on the Spiritual Path* (New York: Bantam Books, Random House, 2001), 98.
2. Macy, *Coming Back to Life: The Updated Guide to "The Work that Reconnects",* 276-278.
3. Gilbert Walking Bull, "Orderly Fashion Prayer," Jon Young, personal communication.
4. Young, *What the Robin Said: How Birds Reveal the Secrets of the Natural World,* 48-79.
5. E. E. Cummings, *Selected Poems,* edited by Richard S. Kennedy (New York: W. W. Norton & Company Ltd, 2007), 167

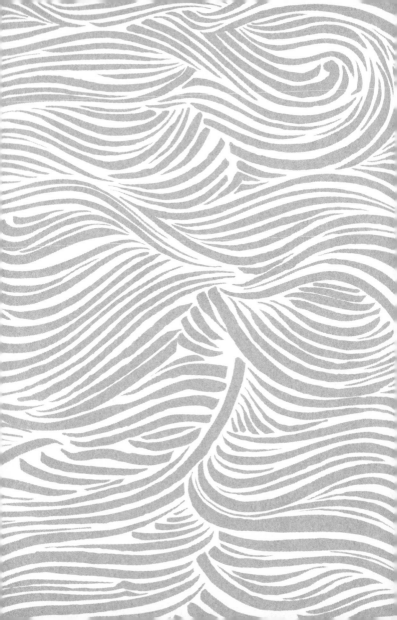

ABOUT THE AUTHOR

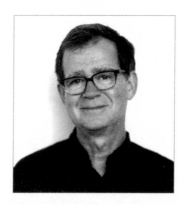

MICHAEL KEARNEY is a physician specializing in hospice and palliative medicine, with over 35 years' experience. He has lived in Ireland, England, France, and Canada before moving to the United States in 2001. He currently lives in Santa Barbara, California, where he is a founding partner of Palliative Care Consultants of Santa Barbara. Michael is married to psychologist, meditation teacher, and author Radhule Weininger, PhD. They teach and write together and share six adult children between them. Additional content related to this book can be found at www.michaelkearneymd.com.

ACKNOWLEDGMENTS

I begin by thanking Radhule, my darling wife and best friend. She has been with me every step of the way—encouraging, challenging, teaching, and inspiring me.

I thank my three beloved daughters, Mary-Anna, Claire, and Ruth, who have given me loving support from afar, including reading the manuscript and offering me helpful feedback. I thank my stepchildren, Joshua, Bella, and Ben, who have been patient and understanding as I have disappeared, again and again, to "work on my book."

I feel so blessed to have had Barbara Gates's warm and bright editorial input during the writing of my book. Again, and again she helped me to find my voice, while always challenging me to think of the reader.

Acknowledgments

I am thankful to Rachel Neumann for opening the publishing door and saying yes to my manuscript. It has been a joy to work with my editor, Jacob Surpin, who has been kind, available, encouraging, and helpful throughout. My sincere thanks to Terri Saul for her art and production direction, and to Jess Morphew for the exquisite cover art design. And a big thank you to Nancy Fish and her team in marketing. Everyone I have met at Parallax has made what seemed like a daunting process easy and enjoyable. I am honored to be part of this community.

In the earliest pages of the book you are introduced to a young man named Ben, who is living, and dying, with cancer. I asked Ben if I could share his story in a book I was writing, adding that I felt he had a lot to teach others. He immediately said yes. He asked me to tell him about the book, which I did. Later, I shared the finished manuscript with his mother, Juanita. I wanted to make sure that she was happy with how I had told her son's story. She took the manuscript to read and we met afterward. She told me that she had wept while reading about Ben. She said she was happy for me to share Ben's story and hoped that it might be a help to others. I am deeply grateful to Ben and Juanita.

I am especially grateful to my mentor and dear friend Joanna Macy. I have learned and continue to learn so much from this huge-hearted, Earth-loving elder. She has been, and continues to be, a huge inspiration to me. Thank you, Joanna, for your encouragement always, and for your beautiful foreword.

I was fortunate to have the opportunity of being mentored by Jon Young during the writing of the book. I have learned so much from Jon about demystifying the practice of nature connection, and making it as accessible as our own backyards. Thank you, Jon.

Even though I never had the opportunity to meet Irish philosopher and poet John Moriarty in person, his thinking, published work, and orally recorded teachings educated and encouraged me to begin writing this book in the first place. I am deeply grateful for the inspiration I have received and continue to receive from this great Celtic bard.

When I told my beloved godmother, Dorothy Cross (Senior), that I was writing a book, she asked, "Is it a big book?" "Yes," I replied (at that time it was more than 180,000 words!) "I think you should write a short book," she said, "No one reads big books anymore." I took your advice, Aunty Dor. Thank you!

There are many others who have helped me by reading the manuscript in its various iterations, and offering me critical feedback and words of encouragement and endorsement: Ed Bastian, Rick Beckett, Robbie Bosnak, Ed Casey, Mario Cepeda, Kathy Corcoran, Dorothy Cross, Antony Farrell, Catherine Gautier, Leslie Gray, Richard Groves, Kurt Goerwitz, Tom

Acknowledgments

Hutchinson, Steve Jacobson, Richard Kearney, Sally Kearney, Carolyn Kenny, Krista Lawlor, Stephen Liben, Teddy Macker, Elaine McCracken, BJ Miller, Thomas Moore, Bal Mount, James Morley, Anne Price, Dave Richo, Souken Danjo, Mary Vachon, and Mary Watkins. My thanks to each of you, and to anyone I have inadvertently missed, please forgive me.

Finally, I want to thank Juliet Spohn-Twomey and Stephanie Glatt, who allowed me to come onto the grounds of La Casa de Maria Retreat and Conference Center in Santa Barbara to write. There I would sit, under the oaks or by the creek. The book is a co-creation with this sacred land and the beings who live there.

DESCENDANTS OF THE EARTH

Descendants of the Earth is a community-based nonprofit organization under the leadership and service of Wolf and Lisa Wahpepah, whose vision is to preserve the integrity of traditional Native American culture for the benefit of all people, while promoting the noncommercialization of Native teachings. Native culture has much to contribute to the environmental restoration of Mother Earth, promoting harmony in interpersonal relationships, and peaceful resolution to larger conflicts that affect the welfare of all people.

CONTACT INFORMATION

Descendants of the Earth,
PO Box 301, Ventura, CA 93002,
United States of America

Phone (office): 805-677-4075

A portion of royalties from the sale of this book
will go to Descendants of the Earth.

RELATED TITLES

Holding Space, Amy Wright Glenn

Love Letter to the Earth, Thich Nhat Hanh

No Mud, No Lotus, Thich Nhat Hanh

Ocean of Insight, Heather Lyn Mann

Pass It On, Joanna Macy

World as Lover, World as Self, Joanna Macy

Zooburbia, Tai Moses

**PARALLAX
PRESS**

Parallax Press is a nonprofit publisher, founded and inspired by Zen Master Thich Nhat Hanh. We publish books on mindfulness in daily life and are committed to making these teachings accessible to everyone and preserving them for future generations. We do this work to alleviate suffering and contribute to a more just and joyful world.

For a copy of the catalog, please contact:

Parallax Press
P.O. Box 7355
Berkeley, CA 94707
parallax.org